ON-CALL
in Trauma and Orthopaedics

Mr Philip S Pastides
FRCS (Tr&Orth) MSc (Orth Eng)

Mr Sanjeeve Sabharwal
FRCS (Tr & Orth) MD(Res) Msc

Mr Khaled M Sarraf
FRCS (Tr&Orth)

Mr Nadeem Mushtaq
MBBS MSc (Orth) FRCS (Tr&Orth)

Foreword by:
Mr P Reilly

Photographs by:
Mr P S Pastides

Series editors:
Mr Arpan S. Tahim
Mr Karl F.B. Payne
Mr Alexander M.C. Goodson

First published in 2018 by Libri Publishing

ISBN 978-1-911450-24-5

Cover and Design by Carnegie Publishing

Printed in the UK by Halstan

Libri Publishing
Brunel House
Volunteer Way
Faringdon
Oxfordshire
SN7 7YR

Tel: +44 (0)845 873 3837

www.libripublishing.co.uk

CONTENTS

ABOUT THE EDITORIAL TEAM

Mr Arpan S Tahim BSc(Hons) MBBS BDS MRCS Med

Specialty Trainee in Oral and Maxillofacial Surgeyr, London Deanery

Mr Karl FB Payne BMedSci(Hons) BMBS BDS MRCS

Specialty Trainee in Oral and Maxillofacial Surgery, West Midlands Deanery

Mr Alexander MC Goodson BSc(Hons) MBBS BDS MRCS DOHNS

Specialty Trainee in Oral and Maxillofacial Surgery, Wales Deanery

ABOUT THE ON-CALL SERIES

The "On-call" series is a unique learning resource consisting of concise, accessible and highly readable books. Authored and edited by a team with a strong focus on medical and surgical education, they have proven to be highly useful both for junior doctors seeking guidance early on in their clinical rotations and for those with more experience who are looking to consolidate and develop their knowledge. Written as "survival guides," each book covers common presentations in the emergency, ward and clinic settings, along with detailed step-by-step descriptions of typical surgical procedures. The attention to hands-on practical advice with easy to follow instructions mean they are the only handbooks that a junior trainee should not be without.

DEDICATION

Pastides

To my fantastic wife Claudia without whose hands, feet and knee this book would not have been possible, and my very loud children Antonia, Thomas and Ellie.

Sabharwal

To my beautiful wife who has supported me through all my endeavours and my wonderful children who make every day more exciting and fun filled.

Sarraf

To my amazing wife Bana, for her endless support in all that I do and my son Karim who has brought infinite joy and love into our life.

Mushtaq

To my beautiful and supportive wife Sandhya and children Imaan, Zayan and Aahil.

ABBREVIATIONS

AP – Anterior-Posterior

ATLS – Advanced Trauma Life Support

BAPRAS – British Assoication of Plastic, Reconstructive and Aesthetic Surgeons

BOA – British Orthopaedic Association

CRT – Capillary refill time

CT – Computer Tomography

DHS – Dynamic Hip Screw

ECG – Electrocardiogram

ED – Emergency department

FBC – Full blood count

G and S – Group and Save

IV – Intravenous

MRI – Magnetic Resonance Imaging

MRSA – Methicillin-resistant Staphylococcus aureus

NICE – National Institute for Health and Care Excellence

NOF – Neck of femur

OPD – Outpatient Department

ORIF – Open reduction internal fixation

POP – Plaster of Paris

RTC – Road Traffic Collision

TCI – To come in

U and Es – Urea and Electrolytes

US – Ultrasonography

VFC – Virtual Fracture Clinic

FOREWORD

It is a pleasure to be asked to write a foreword for this excellent book. It is well conceived and delivered, providing information in an accessible format for junior orthopaedic surgeons on-call. The level of detail is perfect for managing acute patients effectively and also to withstand the cross-examination by the consultant at the next day's trauma meeting! Furthermore its value as a revision aid leading up to the FRCS course should not be overlooked. I congratulate the authors on their work.

Mr Peter Reilly MS FRCS (Orth)

Consultant Orthopaedic Surgeon

INTRODUCTION

Trauma and Orthopaedic surgery is the specialty that manages acute and chronic conditions of the bony skeleton and the soft tissues that are associated with them. Its scope is far reaching which means there is a wide range of traumatic injuries that may present during an on-call shift. Its unpredictability tends to cause anxiety and stress to the on-call orthopaedic doctor. An organised approach to patient assessment and management will help mitigate this.

This book aims to give the junior orthopaedic surgeon an introductory grasp of the specialty whilst also challenging the more experienced orthopaedic trainee to think more holistically about any cases being referred. Using it as a 'survival guide' the reader will learn how to take emergency referrals for patients from the ED, and institute initial management of common orthopaedic presentations before recruiting the help of a senior. The reader will also learn about day-to-day management of in-patients on the ward, as well as dealing with patients in the clinic environment. Finally, practical step-by-step guidance is provided for minor surgical procedures, often performed by the junior orthopaedic surgeon.

This book will serve you well if read prior to starting your first job in orthopaedic surgery, but will also remain a valuable resource on a day-to-day basis as a concise, quick-reference text. From basic clerking, basic classifications, early management, pitfalls and even theatre preparation, we hope that this book will act as a 'senior trauma doctor in your pocket'.

Help is always available; we hope this is your first port of call!

PSP

DISCLAIMER

This book is not a textbook, but a survival guide. All content has been written by the authors and is obtained from reliable sources and based on personal experience. The authors and publisher do not accept responsibility or legal liability for injury or damage to any person as a result of action or refraining from action due to the clinical material within this book. At the time of printing drug doses contained within this book were correct, but it is the reader's responsibility to check up-to-date manufacturer and drug dose safety guidelines.

ESSENTIALS

PATIENTS UNDER YOUR CARE AND PREPARING FOR BEING ON-CALL

As with any acute specialty, the range of patients that may be under your care during the on-call may be both numerous and diverse; children, teenagers, elderly, pre-operative, post-operative, emergency or elective and this list is by no means exhaustive.

It is important not to be overwhelmed by this fact. The truth is that during your on-call shift, most of your patients will be medically stable, recovering from an operation or needing allied professional input (such as physiotherapy or occupational therapy). However, you will also be asked to see a small number of these patients acutely, either upon presentation or in the post-operative environment, who require more urgent management. Rather than feeling worried, enjoy and embrace this opportunity as you may be clerking in an elderly patient one minute and then called to see a child in the cubicle next door.

A lot of anxiety tends to arise amongst junior doctors when they are asked to cover an orthopaedic on-call. Whilst it is likely that, at least for part of your shift, you may be busy, stressed or both, being organised and time-efficient can help in part to alleviate some of these worries.

While preparing for your shift, remember what to take with you

THIS BOOK!!!

Black pen(s)

Black permanent marker pen

Paper to keep a list of admitted/reviewed patients

Mobile phone

Mobile phone charger

Food/drink

TOP TIP:

Remember help is only ever a phone call away; if in doubt ASK FOR HELP!

REFERRALS – WHERE THEY COME FROM AND HOW TO ACCEPT THEM

ESSENTIALS

Patients tend to be referred to the Trauma and Orthopaedic services from four main sources:

- Via the Emergency Department.
- Via a GP in the community.
- Via other medical teams within the hospital.
- Via your own team from clinic.

You should also be aware that if you are working in a specialised unit, such as paediatrics or hands, then referrals may also come from other hospitals.

The key is to take a history from the person referring as well as their examination and/or radiographic findings if possible. You should also ask them what THEY think the diagnosis is or alternatively what their concerns are.

Be courteous to all referring clinicians. There are, albeit infrequent, complaints where the on-call doctor was rude, unhelpful or dismissive over the telephone while discussing potential referrals. There are times when you will be struggling to deal with the workload and working hard to manage several different concurrent problems. In these situations, try to put yourself in the referrer's shoes. They are NOT specialists in trauma or orthopaedics and frequently they do NOT have access to the radiographs or investigations. It may also involve a patient that they saw several days ago and whose test result they have only just received. They will be genuinely concerned for their patient and similar to yourself will be taking time out of their own busy workload to ask for your opinion and, more importantly, your help with a situation they are unable to manage. If you are unsure whether a patient needs to be seen then ask your senior colleague for advice or, to be safe and helpful, let the patient come as a referral and assess them yourself or with your senior.

A classic, recurring example is a GP trying to refer a possible septic joint. A GP will be unable to perform immediate blood tests or radiographs and may only be able to tell you that a patient has a hot and painful joint with a low grade temperature. It is your role in the orthopaedic department to help your community colleagues and exclude emergency conditions.

ADMISSIONS

Regardless of where patients are referred from, if you are admitting them to the ward, all assessments will start with taking a full history. This will be very similar to the standard format of history taking you are familiar with, but focusing on a few key additions. Following this, you will need to carry out your examination of the affected region.

ESSENTIALS

HISTORY

BACKGROUND

- Age of patient.
- Dominance of limb.
- Occupation.

PRESENTING COMPLAINT

Mechanism of injury:

- Fall
    - Mechanical (e.g. a trip).
    - Non-mechanical (e.g. fainting episode).
    - Height from which fall occurred.
- Slip
    - What broke the fall (e.g. landed on bottom, on an outstretched limb).
- Road Traffic Collision (RTC)
    - Were they a pedestrian or a driver?
    - Motor vehicle or bicycle or motorbike?
    - How violent was the impact?
        - Did the vehicle air bags deploy in the car?
        - Did they need to be extricated from the vehicle?

Have they mobilised since the event?

Where is the pain?

How severe is the pain?

Was there any blood at the scene?

Any numbness/tingling in any limb?

Specifically for back injuries:
- Is there any numbness or reduced sensation around back passage?
- Do they have any problems passing urine or opening their bowels?

Any other injuries?

PAST MEDICAL HISTORY
Any other medical problems
Previous limb injuries or fractures

DRUG HISTORY
List and doses of medications
Specifically ask for use of anticoagulant and anti-platelet agents

SOCIAL HISTORY
Smoking history and alcohol history
Housing situation – house/flat

Are there stairs in or to the property? If so, how many?
- Does the property have an elevator?
- Is there a toilet downstairs?

Who lives with them?
- Can they look after them upon discharge?

How do they normally walk?
- Can they walk both inside and outside of the house?
- How far and what stops them walking further?
- Do they use any walking aids? If so what (stick, zimmer frame, wheelchair)?

Do they drive?

EXAMINATION
You should follow the basic principles: LOOK, FEEL, MOVE. In trauma, we tend to either already have a diagnosis from the ED if it has been referred to us, or have reviewed the radiographs if they have presented through fracture clinic.

It will be difficult to ask them to move the fractured limb or bone but remember to assess function of the joint above and below the injured region.

Always assess the neurovascular status distal to the zone of injury.

NEUROVASCULAR ASSESSMENT

It is important to remember that any bony injury will also have a soft tissue component to it as well. This may present purely as bruising or a haematoma, however it is important to assess the function of the nerves and blood vessels as a result of the trauma. It is also important to remember that a nerve has both a sensory and a motor function. Both may be difficult to assess due to pain, especially the motor function, however efforts should be made to examine and document this. This is crucial when we are dealing with a displaced fracture that we will be reducing acutely; function before and after reduction MUST be documented.

As a rule of thumb, function of the nerve at the most distal level to the injury implies that the nerve is still functional.

In this section we describe a few key screening tests that can be performed by the bedside to assess function of the key upper and lower limb nerves. If there is any concern, then a more thorough and detailed examination should be performed, documented and seniors alerted.

UPPER LIMB

NEUROLOGICAL SCREEN

There are 5 main nerves to assess during this examination. It is best to assess them with the arm held in the anatomical position (i.e. the palm is facing forwards)

- Axillary nerve (Figure 1.1)
- Musculocutaneous nerve
    - Sensory: lateral aspect forearm
    - Motor: elbow flexion and supination
- Radial nerve (Figure 1.2)
- Ulna nerve (Figure 1.3)
- Median nerve (Figure 1.4)

VASCULAR SCREEN

To begin, simply assess capillary refill time by pressing on the nail bed for 5 seconds. The colour should return within 2–3 seconds. The radial and ulna pulses should also be assessed as shown in Figure 1.5.

ESSENTIALS

ESSENTIALS

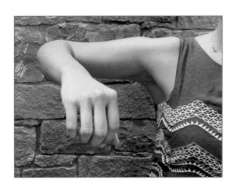

Figure 1.1.

- *Axillary nerve*
- *Sensory: over regimental patch area*
- *Motor: shoulder abduction*

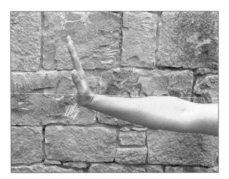

Figure 1.2.

- *Radial nerve*
- *Sensory: skin overlying the first webspace of dorsum hand*
- *Motor: wrist and finger extension*

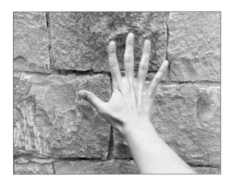

Figure 1.3.

- *Ulna nerve*
- *Sensory: skin overlying the little finger and ulna half of ring finger*
- *Motor: finger abduction*

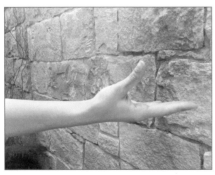

Figure 1.4.

- *Median nerve*
- *Sensory: skin overlying the thumb, index, middle and radial half of ring fingers*
- *Motor: flexion of the thumb*

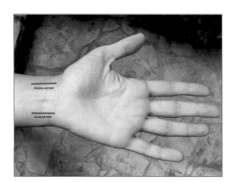

Figure 1.5.

- *Distal pulses (radial and ulna) at the wrist*

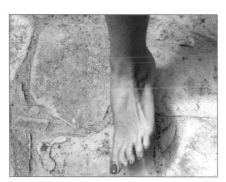

Figure 1.6.

- *Superficial peroneal nerve*
- *Sensory: Dorsum of the foot (except first webspace)*
- *Motor: eversion of the ankle*

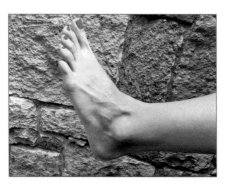

Figure 1.7.

- *Deep peroneal nerve*
- *Sensory: skin overlying the first webspace dorsum of the foot*
- *Motor: dorsiflexion of the ankle and toes*

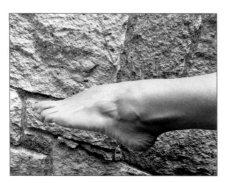

Figure 1.8.

- *Tibial Nerve*
- *Sensory: skin overlying the sole of the foot*
- *Motor: Plantarflexion at the ankle*

ESSENTIALS

LOWER LIMB

NEUROLOGICAL SCREEN

The 3 important nerves that are assessed in this examination are the femoral, the common peroneal and tibial nerves. The two latter nerves arise from the sciatic nerve.

- Femoral nerve
    - Sensory: anteromedial thigh
    - Motor: hip flexion and knee extension
- Common peroneal nerve – superficial branch (Figure 1.6)
- Common peroneal nerve – deep branch (Figure 1.7)
- Tibial nerve (Figure 1.8)

VASCULAR SCREEN

Assess capillary refill time by pressing on the nail bed for 5 seconds. The colour should return within 2–3 seconds. The pulses to palpate are the popliteal, dorsalis pedis and posterior tibialis (Figure 1.9). Remember that the popliteal artery is a deep structure and can be difficult to feel.

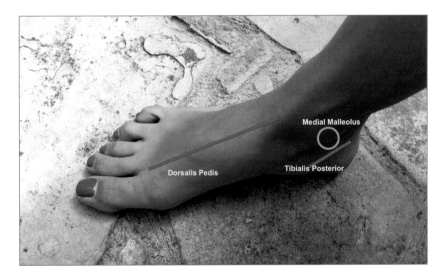

Figure 1.9.
- *Dorsalis pedis artery: felt just proximal to the first webspace*
- *Posterior tibialis artery: medial ankle, midway point between the medial malleolus and the calcaneus*

TOP TIP:

If the patient had no immediate neurovascular deficit but over the next few hours starts to develop positive signs, always think to split any plaster and wool bandages they may have to expose the underlying skin. DO NOT worry about losing reduction of an underlying fracture. If there is any concern about compartment syndrome, call your senior immediately! (see page 26)

ESSENTIALS

A NOTE ON ADMISSIONS FROM FRACTURE OR OUTPATIENTS CLINIC

When clerking patients from a clinic, always ask the senior doctor who is requesting the admission whether the patient is to be admitted on the day or discharged home and contacted once a slot is identified on a suitable trauma theatre list. If they are to be discharged, ensure:

- You have taken a contact number for the patient.
- The patient has been consented.
- The consent form and your clerking is FILED in the notes.
- Any necessary blood tests, ECG and MRSA swabs (if necessary) have been requested.
- The notes have been placed somewhere secure so they can be found on the day (for example most hospitals have a box/tray in theatre where these notes are placed in order to ensure that they are accessible).
- Document in the notes which senior doctor has decided that this patient needs an operation.

CLASSIFICATIONS OF COMMON FRACTURES

The role of any classification system is to provide a uniform language of communication between treating clinicians, with an aim of providing treatment options, rehabilitation programs and prognosis of outcomes. You will also regularly be asked to classify the common fractures during fracture clinics, trauma meetings and whilst on-call so it is important to become familiar with them. As well as allowing you to impress your colleagues, a working knowledge of these classifications will leave you better placed to have a discussion with the patient about treatment options.

Many classification systems are quite complex and detailed and certainly beyond the scope of this book but as a general rule, as the grade of the fracture increases, the treatment becomes more difficult and the outcome becomes less predictable.

These are the most widely used systems for each of the common injuries below:

- Intracapsular Neck of Femur fractures – *Garden Classification.*
- Fractures around Proximal Femur.
- Fractures around Tibial Plateau – *Schatzker Classification.*
- Lateral Malleolar fractures – *Weber Classification.*
- Supracondylar Paediatric Elbow fractures – *Gartland Classification.*
- Paediatric Epiphyseal fractures – *Salter-Harris Classification.*
- *Gustilo Anderson open fracture Classification.*

GARDEN CLASSIFICATION – INTRACAPSULAR NECK OF FEMUR FRACTURE

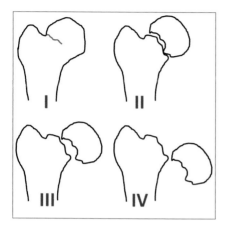

Figure 1.10 Garden Classification.

Grade I	Incomplete fracture	Fixation / conservative
Grade II	Undisplaced complete fracture	Fixation
Grade III	Partially displaced fracture	Replacement (hemiarthroplasty)
Grade IV	Completely displaced fracture	Replacement (hemiarthroplasty)

A useful way to remember this is using the mnemonic '*Grade 1, 2 Screw Grade 3, 4 Austin Moore*' (which is an old type of hemiarthroplasty). This means that grade 1 and 2 fractures are likely to require fixation using a dynamic hip screw, whereas higher grade fractures will require hemiarthroplasties.

TOP TIP

There is a recent trend to perform Total Hip Replacements (THR) rather than a hemiarthroplasty in active patients for Grade III and IV (NICE Guidelines).

ESSENTIALS

FRACTURE AROUND PROXIMAL FEMUR

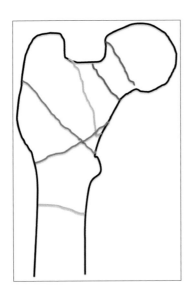

Figure 1.11. Fractures around Proximal Femur.

Red	Subcapital fracture	
Green	Transcervical fracture	Intracapsular
Purple	Basocervical fracture	
Blue	Intertrochanteric fracture	Extracapsular
Fuschia	Reverse Oblique	
Orange	Subtrochanteric	Subtrochanteric

SCHATZKER CLASSIFICATION – FRACTURES AROUND TIBIAL PLATEAU

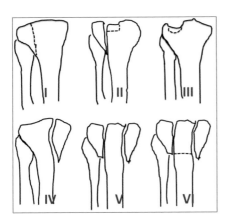

Figure 1.12. Schatzker Classification.

Type I	Lateral plateau split
Type II	Lateral plateau split and depression of articular surface
Type III	Lateral plateau articular depression
Type IV	Medial plateau fracture
Type V	Bicondylar fracture
Type VI	Fracture with metaphyseal component

A useful mnemonic for remembering Type I to III is to think of them in terms of a romantic break up:

First you SPLIT up

Then you have SPLIT up and are DEPRESSED

Then you are over the split but are still DEPRESSED

WEBER CLASSIFICATION – LATERAL MALLEOLAR FRACTURES

Figure 1.13. Weber Classification.

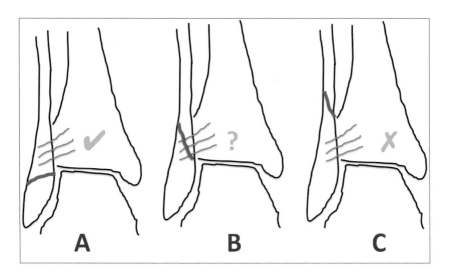

Weber A	Fracture below level of syndesmosis	Syndesmosis intact
Weber B	Fracture at level of syndesmosis	Syndesmosis possibly intact
Weber C	Fracture above the syndesmosis	Syndesmosis ruptured

ESSENTIALS

GARTLAND CLASSIFICATION – SUPRACONDYLAR PAEDIATRIC ELBOW FRACTURES

Figure 1.14. Gartland Classification.

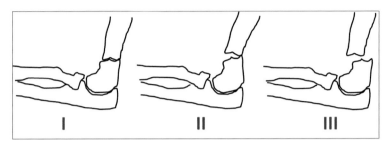

Gartland I	Undisplaced fracture
Gartland II	Minimally displaced fracture with an intact posterior periosteal hinge
Gartland III	Displaced fracture

SALTER-HARRIS CLASSIFICATION – PAEDIATRIC EPIPHYSEAL FRACTURES

Figure 1.15. Salter-Harris Classification.

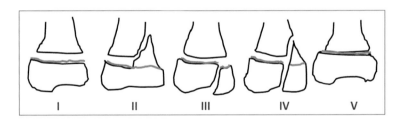

Type I	**S** eparation	Separation of epiphysis and physis
Type II	**A** bove	Fracture traverses physis and metaphysis
Type III	**L** ower	Fracture involving physis and epiphysis only
Type IV	**T** hrough	Fracture involves physis, epiphysis and metaphysis
Type V	**R** ammed	Impaction of epiphysis and physis

These fractures can be recalled as the first letters (almost) spell its eponymous name: S-A-L-T-R (see above table)

GUSTILO ANDERSON OPEN FRACTURE CLASSIFICATION

This system is the most commonly used classification system for open fractures. It combines the amount of energy, extent of soft-tissue injury and the extent of contamination of the wound.

1	Low energy, simple fracture, <1cm wound size, clean wound, local soft tissue coverage available, no neurovascular compromise
2	Moderate energy, moderate severity fracture, >1cm <10cm wound size, moderate contamination, local soft tissue coverage available, no neurovascular compromise
3A	High-energy, severe fracture pattern, >10cm wound , extensive contamination, periosteal stripping, local soft tissue coverage available, no neurovascular compromise
3B	High-energy, severe fracture pattern, >10cm wound , extensive contamination, periosteal stripping, requires free tissue or rotational flap coverage, no neurovascular compromise
3C	High-energy, severe fracture pattern, >10cm wound , extensive contamination, periosteal stripping, requires free tissue or rotational flap coverage, arterial damage that requires repair/reconstruction

Please note it is used as a pre-operative classification system but in its original description, it was used to classify the injuries POST surgical debridement; a small puncture wound may seem to be a grade 1, however after debridement, the extent of degloving may be so severe that it progresses to a more severe grade.

ESSENTIALS

THE TRAUMA MEETING

The trauma and orthopaedic team typically meet every morning to discuss the referrals over the previous 24 hours and the pending trauma cases, in what is colloquially known as 'the trauma meeting'. Often, one of your senior colleagues will have reviewed the patients prior to the meeting and presented the histories prior to discussing ongoing management. However, occasionally this may be your responsibility. Either way, active participation and engagement in this meeting is vital to ensure a smooth handover and no delays to the trauma theatre list.

Also remember that you may have handed over or been handed over by the departing on-call shift several tasks to do for the admitted patients, such as check blood results, review ECGs etc. Please make sure that these tasks have been performed as it may lead to delays or even cancellation of theatre cases which will ultimately be detrimental for patient care.

PRE TRAUMA MEETING ESSENTIALS

These meetings will vary slightly between departments but overall, it is important to ensure that:

- All patients admitted/reviewed are listed on an appropriate admissions database so they can be discussed.
- All patients who require surgery are listed on the trauma theatre board.
- A trauma theatre list for the day has been submitted in theatres.
- All patients on the trauma list are marked, consented and fasted.
- All patients have the appropriate blood tests.
- Theatre and anaesthetic staff are aware of the first patient on the list.
- You are aware of the important blood results for the pre-operative patients and those admitted during the on-call take.

THE TRAUMA MEETING

If asked to present at the trauma meeting, aim to keep your case summaries succinct and to the point. You must

1. Get the key parts of the history/past medical history across in a condensed fashion.
2. Focus on the actual injury the patient has sustained.
3. If confident, you could then explain what procedure the patient has been listed for.
4. Outline the results of pre-operative investigations to ensure they are suitable.

FOR EXAMPLE

'An 86-year-old lady was admitted following a mechanical fall at home, when she tripped on a carpet. She suffers with hypertension and mild asthma. She takes inhalers on a prn basis. She lives alone in a ground floor flat and mobilises with a stick. She has carers once a day and her daughter visits a couple of times a week and brings her shopping. She presented via ED with a painful left hip and the leg was shortened and externally rotated. She had no neurovascular deficit. Radiographs revealed an intertrochanteric neck of femur fracture. Her pre-operative haemoglobin is 10.8 and she has normal renal function. She has 2 valid Group and Save samples. She is fasted, marked and consented for a dynamic hip screw'.

Presenting in the above manner tells the trauma team all the information that they need and also shows a complete and perfectly executed pre-operative plan. You could even practice your case presentation with a senior colleague before the meeting to make sure the plan and terminology is correct.

ESSENTIALS

SHOULD I ADMIT THIS PATIENT?

This is a key question for an on-call doctor, especially one with limited experience in trauma and orthopaedics. It is important to use both your clinical judgment and also common sense to try and answer it. Should you feel that they need admission then either contact your senior for advice or admit them for a later senior review and potential discharge. You must be safe and act in what you feel is the patient's best interest.

Below is a 9-point list of issues that you might consider before deciding:

1. **Lower leg trauma that means the patient is unable or unsafe to be discharged home.** This includes neck of femur fractures, long bone fractures that require obvious surgery, but also consider ankle fractures in patients who are unsafe on crutches or live alone with no one to look after them at home.

2. **Elderly patients with trauma that may or may not require surgery but will be seriously handicapped should they be discharged.** An example includes a proximal humerus fracture in an elderly patient.

3. **Pain.** If a patient, irrespective of age, is in severe pain then they should be admitted for analgesia and reassessment.

4. **Suspected causes of non-accidental trauma.** Be alert as this can affect patients of any age.

5. **Any injury with an associated neurological or vascular injury.** It may be associated with a displaced fracture and resolved following reduction. However, it may be worth keeping them for observation. Discuss with your senior if unsure.

6. **Dislocated joints**. Do not send patients home if they have joints (any joint, big or small) that are dislocated.

7. **Anyone who you think is likely to need an operation AND there is space on the trauma list the next day.** This illustrates why it is worth knowing what cases are pending/listed for the next day and will help facilitate efficient case flow.

8. **Any case of a suspected septic joint** (native or prosthetic).

9. **Anyone that YOU are concerned about for whatever reason.**

CAN I SAFELY SEND THE PATIENT HOME?

This is another important question, which requires your clinical judgment and common sense. For example, if the trauma list is already full with more urgent cases, then it is potentially acceptable to send patients home and to bring them back at a later date. They must fulfill the following criteria:

1. They are comfortable.

2. They have someone with them to look after them.

3. They are neurovascularly intact.

4. They have low energy injuries.

If you have made the decision to discharge a patient home, there are some key practicalities to address:

- You must ensure that you have a reliable means by which to contact them (at least one, ideally two, working telephone numbers).

- You should provide them with contact details to use in case of deterioration.

- You must ensure they have appropriate follow up, either with their GP, fracture clinic or elsewhere.

- If in doubt of the need for surgery, you can always send the patient home and contact them after the trauma meeting. If you keep them starved, then they may still be able to have their operation should there be space on the trauma list.

DISABLING, LIMB OR LIFE-THREATENING CONDITIONS

Although rare, there are several conditions that may threaten life or have the potential for profound morbidity. It is important that the on-call trauma and orthopaedic doctor is able to recognize these injuries and alert their relevant senior.

These injuries include:

- Pelvic fractures.
- Open fractures.
- Compartment syndrome.
- Cauda equina syndrome.

PELVIC FRACTURES

Almost all these cases are related to trauma, usually road traffic collisions (driver or pedestrian) or falls from heights. However the elderly patient with osteoporotic bone may have simply fallen from standing and suffered pelvic injuries.

RADIOLOGICAL ASSESSMENT

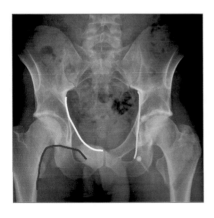

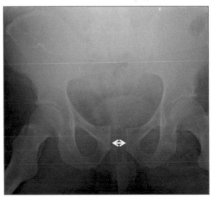

Figure 2.1.

- *Blue line: Shenton's line*
- *Yellow line: Ilioischial line*
- *White line: Iliopectineal line*

Figure 2.2. Pelvic fracture showing widening of the pubic symphysis.

EMERGENCY DEPARTMENT

KEY POINTS – HISTORY

What was the mechanism of injury?

What medications they are on, in particular anticoagulants

KEY POINTS – CLINICAL ASSESSMENT

Are there any signs of haemodynamic instability – if so, assume there is a pelvic injury until it is excluded

Is there tenderness over pelvis?

Is there a leg length discrepancy/deformity?

Bruising or bleeding in the perineal or genital region?

MANAGEMENT

- These patients may have significant injuries and as such should be managed using ATLS guidelines.
- Most patients will attend with a pelvic binder in situ if such an injury is suspected; if not in place but a pelvic injury is suspected, place one immediately.
- Any haemodynamic instability is due to bleeding (usually venous) that occurs as a result of the disruption of the pelvic bones rupturing the vascular plexus. It is imperative that patients are resuscitated with blood products rather than crystalloid/colloid fluids.
- The key is to try and stem the haemorrhage. Sometimes this is achieved simply with the application of a pelvic binder and administration of blood and clotting factors. Occasionally interventional radiology and embolization can be attempted or, if the patient is very unstable, then pelvic packing with or without application of a pelvic external fixator may be employed.

TOP TIP

If in doubt, always get a CT scan of the pelvis in order to exclude a pelvic injury and ALWAYS alert your senior early if such a patient presents to your hospital.

OPEN FRACTURES

When describing bony injuries, remember that an open fracture is the direct communication of the **fracture haematoma** and the outside world, **NOT** only the bone itself. They occur after direct or indirect trauma to the affected limb and the tibia is the most common site of injury.

KEY POINTS – HISTORY

What was the mechanism of injury?

Where did the injury occur?

- Indoors/outdoors/urban/rural setting

What is the drug and allergy history?

When was the last time the patient ate or drank?

Is there any numbness or tingling in the digits distal to the fracture site?

KEY POINTS – CLINICAL ASSESSMENT

Is there any limb swelling or deformity?

Assess the limb for neurovascular compromise.

Check capillary refill time distal to the fracture.

Injuries can be classified by the **Gustilo Anderson open fracture classification** system.

MANAGEMENT

- As per ATLS guidelines.
- If there is an obvious deformity and neurovascular compromise, the limb needs to be IMMEDIATELY realigned. This is best done under sedation and the senior ED doctors or anaesthetic team will be able to assist you. YOU SHOULD NOT WAIT FOR A RADIOGRAPH!
- In those cases with no evidence of neurovascular compromise:
    - Apply saline soaked gauze over wound.
    - Start antibiotics (typically co-amoxiclav OR clindamycin if penicillin allergic).
    - Establish tetanus status and deliver booster if the patient is not up to date.
    - Immobilise the limb in a plaster cast.

EMERGENCY DEPARTMENT

- Admit the patient, elevate limb and monitor.
- Alert your senior colleague. Many cases are now managed in combined orthopaedic/plastic units rather than by orthopaedic teams in isolation and thus the patient may need to be transferred out to another hospital.

TOP TIP

If you suspect that the bleeding is coming from a haematoma close to the fracture site, treat it as an open fracture.

COMPARTMENT SYNDROME

This is an uncommon condition that occurs when the pressure within a myofascial compartment rises to such a level that it decreases perfusion of the structures within and subsequently distally to it. It may lead to irreversible muscle and nerve damage. They arise after direct or indirect trauma to a limb, with or without an underlying fracture. The incidence is higher in CLOSED fractures rather than open fractures however the index of suspicion with open fractures should also be extremely high.

KEY POINTS – HISTORY

The mechanism of injury and the degree of pain are important to consider. It is useful to work out whether:

- PAIN is the main clinical sign of this condition.
- PAIN that is out of proportion to the injury.
- PAIN at rest and worse on passive stretching of the muscle within the affected limb compartment.

KEY POINTS – CLINICAL ASSESSMENT

Is the pain worse on passive stretching of the muscle within the limb compartment?

Is there swelling in the compartment which is tense on palpation? Classically it is described as 'woody hard' but this may be a late sign.

Neurovascular compromise needs to be monitored closely but remember **do not wait until a neurovascular deficit has developed as this is a late and poor prognostic indicator.**

MANAGEMENT

- Give the patient some strong analgesia.
- Expose the skin of the affected limb completely. This includes removing bandaging, plaster backslab and wool from the affected limb.
- If there is an underlying open fracture, keep a small adhesive dressing over the wound but make sure it is not circumferentially applied.
- Elevate the limb to above the level of the patient's heart.
- YOU should personally reassess the patient every 15 minutes and if no improvement in symptoms, alert your senior IMMEDIATELY.
- The only treatment for compartment syndrome is a fasciotomy to release the pressure within the myofascial compartment. This involves making skin incisions over the muscle compartments and then releasing the fascia overlying those muscles. This reduces the pressure within that compartment, restoring the blood and oxygen supply to the soft tissues.

EMERGENCY DEPARTMENT

TOP TIPS

Compartment syndrome is a **CLINICAL** diagnosis and if you suspect it, alert your seniors. However some departments may have pressure gauge monitors that can measure the pressure within the myofascial compartment. This can be then used to measure the so-called Delta Pressure. This is the patient's diastolic blood pressure (DBP), minus the intra-compartmental pressure (ICP). If the difference is less than 30mmHg, then the patient should proceed to have a fasciotomy.

If in any doubt call your senior immediately – DO NOT wait until the morning ward round.

CAUDA EQUINA SYNDROME

Cauda equina syndrome is a rare and severe type of spinal stenosis where all of the nerves in the lower back suddenly become severely compressed. The signs and symptoms are explained by understanding the anatomical principle that the bundle of nerves and roots continue below the level where the spinal cord ends (around the L1 vertebra). These are called the cauda equine (horse's tail). There may be a traumatic cause for this syndrome, but it can also occur due to intervertebral disc herniation, tumours or infection.

KEY POINTS – HISTORY

It is important to distinguish between a nerve root impingement (e.g. due to a disc prolapse/sciatica) and cauda equina.

If there was a traumatic presentation, what was the mechanism of injury and are they in pain?

Is there numbness/tingling/loss of sensation down wither or both legs or around the perineal area?

Is there urinary or faecal incontinence?

How long have these symptoms been present for?

KEY POINTS – CLINICAL ASSESSMENT

Conduct a full neurological assessment of BOTH lower legs.

Assess sensory loss around the rectum – light touch and pin prick (blunted needle).

PERFORM A DIGITAL RECTAL EXAMINATION – VERY IMPORTANT
- Can they feel and squeeze your finger in their rectum?
- Is the sphincter tone (strength) normal?

MANAGEMENT
- If you suspect cauda equina, alert your senior immediately!
- During normal working hours, you may be able to get an urgent MRI scan but do not wait for a scan to seek help.
- Most hospitals have a dedicated regional neurosurgical centre that you can contact for advice or transfer of the patient if needed.

TOP TIPS

Inserting a urinary catheter is a sensitive way to assess sensation of the urogenital system. Ask the patient if they can feel the catheter being inserted and also, once within the bladder, gently tug on it so the balloon engages with the bladder neck. This is called the 'tug test'.

UPPER LIMB

CLAVICLE FRACTURES

BACKGROUND

These injuries usually occur as a result of a fall onto an outstretched arm or a direct blow to the shoulder. They most commonly affect the middle third of the clavicle (approximately 80%). Lateral third fractures are less common (approximately 15%) but more commonly need surgery, especially if they are comminuted as these are associated with a higher non-union rate. Medial third fractures are the least common type of clavicle fracture (approximately 5%) – but have the potential to compromise the bronchial tree and great vessels.

RADIOLOGICAL ASSESSMENT

Three radiographic views should be obtained; an AP view, a 45° caudal tilt (to assess for AP shortening) and a 15° cephalic tilt (to look for superior/inferior displacement).

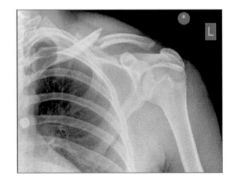

KEY POINTS – HISTORY

In addition to the mechanism of injury, remember to ask about limb dominance and occupation as this may impact on treatment options.

Figure 2.3. AP radiograph showing a displaced midshaft clavicle fracture.

Is there a smoking history – this will impair bone healing.

Ask about numbness/altered sensation/weakness in affected arm.

KEY POINTS – CLINICAL ASSESSMENT

Inspect for any open wounds (any evidence of an open wound requires following the open wound management protocols as per the BOA/BAPRAS guidelines).

The fractured end may tent the skin and cause pressure necrosis, or occasionally actually pierce the skin.

Conduct a full neurovascular assessment of the upper limb.

EMERGENCY DEPARTMENT

MANAGEMENT

- Give appropriate analgesia.
- Place the patient in a broad arm sling or a poly-sling (if available) for comfort. A simple collar and cuff is NOT advisable for clavicle fractures as it may cause more displacement of the fracture.
- Most clavicle fractures can be managed non-operatively and thus can be sent home and discussed in the morning trauma meeting. There are a few indications for operative management to be aware of and the following cases should usually be escalated to a senior straight away:
  - Open fracture, or severe tenting of the skin.
  - Neurovascular injury.
  - Poly-trauma patient.
  - Posteriorly displaced medial third fracture.

Other indications include:
- Shortening of fracture > 2 cm.
- Distal (lateral) third fractures.

EMERGENCY DEPARTMENT

TOP TIPS

If a patient has an extremely painful and tender distal third of clavicle but the x-rays appear normal then consider an injury to the acromio-clavicular joint (ACJ). These injuries are normally obvious due to displacement of the end of the clavicle relative to the acromion, however for the milder ACJ injuries they may be more difficult to spot.

SHOULDER DISLOCATION

BACKGROUND

The vast majority of these injuries are anterior shoulder dislocations (95% of cases) and are caused by a direct force on the arm. Posterior shoulder dislocation, which represent 5% of cases are caused by an axial force through an internally rotated and adducted shoulder. They often occur during epileptic seizures and electrocution. Inferior shoulder dislocation (Luxatio Erecta) occurs in less than 1% of cases where there is hyper-abduction of the shoulder (e.g. falling from a height and trying to hang on to something to stop you falling).

RADIOLOGICAL ASSESSMENT

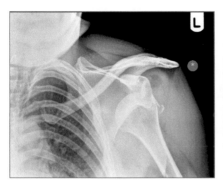

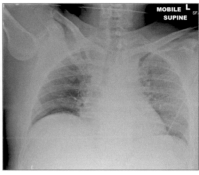

Figure 2.4. Anterior shoulder dislocation.

Figure 2.5. Inferior dislocation of the right shoulder.

EMERGENCY DEPARTMENT

An AP, a scapular Y (a radiograph with the glenoid looking straight on) and an axillary view (a radiograph taken through the armpit) are useful to confirm your diagnosis. The latter is very important in equivocal cases so do not hesitate to send the patient back to the radiology department to obtain the view if it was not performed.

An anterior dislocation is usually quite easy to diagnose on an x-ray (Figure 2.4), however a posterior dislocation is commonly missed on an AP x-ray despite the pathognomonic 'light-bulb' appearance that is often described. If you can't get an axillary view because of discomfort to the patient, request a Velpeau view. Here the patient is leaning backwards at 30° with their arm in a sling and the x-ray beam is placed over the shoulder, with the cassette directly below.

When assessing the x-rays, look very carefully for any fractures. If you are not sure ask a senior to review the x-rays. In some cases a CT scan may be required, as guided by your senior.

KEY POINTS – HISTORY

Establish the mechanism of injury.

Check to see whether the patient is experiencing any numbness, paraesthesia or weakness on the affected side.

Determine whether this is a first episode as recurrent instability has implications for long-term management.

KEY POINTS – ASSESSMENT

A full neurological assessment of the affected limb is required. This should be performed and documented, before and after any attempted reduction of the shoulder.

Assessment of the axillary nerve should be performed. Often it is difficult to assess motor function because of pain, however sensory assessment over the regimental patch must be done.

With each type of dislocation, the arm tends to be held in a specific position:

Anterior: abduction and external rotation.

Posterior: adduction and internal rotation.

Inferior: arm overhead with shoulder in full abduction and elbow flexed.

MANAGEMENT

- Analgesia and sedation should be administered under the supervision of a competent doctor and a nurse. See page 119 for reduction techniques of the shoulder.
- Following a reduction, place the arm in a broad arm sling or a poly-sling. Reassess and document the neurovascular status of the limb. If there is any new abnormality that has developed post reduction you must inform your senior immediately.
- Obtain a post-reduction radiograph in at least two views to confirm a successful reduction.
- For patients who have a successful reduction in ED it is acceptable to discharge them home with follow up in fracture clinic in a week.
- In younger patients in particular, after a traumatic dislocation of the shoulder there is an increased and significant risk of further instability. This group should be discussed in the trauma meeting.

> **TOP TIP**
>
> A good screening tool to assess whether the shoulder is dislocated or not is to ask the patient to touch the tip of the uninjured shoulder with the fingers of the injured shoulder. If they cannot do that then have a high index of suspicion!
>
> If there is a fracture of the proximal humerus (displaced/un-displaced) associated with the dislocation inform your senior immediately. These dislocations should be reduced under general anaesthesia.

PROXIMAL HUMERUS FRACTURE

BACKGROUND

This normally involves a fall onto an outstretched hand in an elderly patient. Fractures in younger patients are seen more with high-energy injuries.

RADIOLOGICAL ASSESSMENT

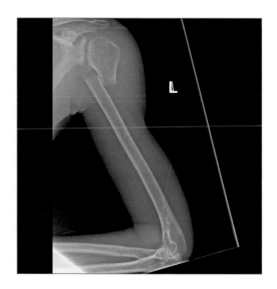

Figure 2.6. AP view of proximal humerus fracture.

EMERGENCY DEPARTMENT

Make sure there are two radiographic views (AP + scapular Y or axillary). This is important to better assess the fracture as well as rule out a fracture dislocation.

KEY POINTS – HISTORY

In addition to the mechanism of injury, remember to ask about limb dominance and occupation as this may impact on treatment options.

Is there a smoking history?

Ask about numbness/altered sensation/weakness in affected arm.

KEY POINTS – CLINICAL ASSESSMENT

It is important to assess the axillary nerve, especially the sensation in regimental patch on arm (lateral aspect of upper arm). The motor function of the deltoid will be difficult to assess due to the injury.

Conduct vascular screen in the limb.

MANAGEMENT

- Make sure there are no other concomitant injuries to the cervical spine or ipsilateral limb (particularly in a high-energy injury).
- Analgesia.
- Immobilise the patient in a collar and cuff or a poly-sling.
- The vast majority of minimally displaced fractures and fractures in the very elderly can be managed conservatively. These patients can be discharged home with outpatient follow up in the fracture clinic in a week. Ensure that these patients have enough analgesia to take home with them.
- For displaced or multi-fragmentary fractures, particularly in patients under the age of 70, there is a growing trend for surgical treatment. Safe and ambulatory patients could go home and be brought back after discussion in the trauma meeting. They may require a CT scan which can be arranged either the following day or on an outpatient basis.
- If there is a fracture of the proximal humerus with a dislocation of the glenohumeral joint, this needs to be admitted for reduction the following day if neurovascularly intact or overnight if compromised.

TOP TIPS

Do not get caught out missing a posterior fracture dislocation of the proximal humerus. If there is a suspicion of such an injury have a low threshold for discussing it with your senior. Occasionally a CT scan is warranted.

As a rule of thumb, never attempt to reduce a fracture dislocation of the proximal humerus in the casualty department.

HUMERAL SHAFT FRACTURES

BACKGROUND

Most commonly occur as a result of direct trauma to the upper limb, characteristically resulting in a transverse fracture. Torsional injuries result in a spiral fracture.

RADIOLOGICAL ASSESSMENT

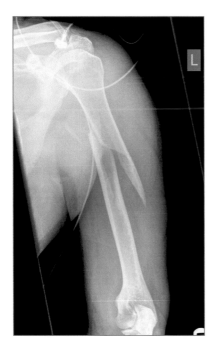

Figure 2.7. AP view demonstrating a spiral fracture of the humeral mid shaft.

EMERGENCY DEPARTMENT

AP and lateral x-rays are required. The fracture is described as proximal, middle or distal third. Ensure that x-rays include the shoulder and elbow joint as there can be extension of the fracture into these joints or a concomitant injury.

KEY POINTS – HISTORY

In addition to the mechanism of injury, remember to ask about limb dominance and occupation as this may impact on treatment options.

It there a smoking history?

Ask about numbness/altered sensation/weakness in affected arm.

KEY POINTS – CLINICAL ASSESSMENT

Inspect for any open wounds.

Examination of the radial nerve is very important in these injuries due to the nature of its anatomical course. It crosses from the posterior compartment to the anterior compartment of the upper limb about 14cm proximal to the lateral epicondyle, in the distal third of the humerus. Therefore, there is a high risk of nerve injury with these fractures. A spiral fracture of the distal 1/3 is commonly associated with a radial nerve neuropraxia; these are called Holstein-Lewis fractures.

MANAGEMENT

- Early immobilisation with a low collar and cuff (wrist at the level of the umbilicus) along with analgesia are important for patient comfort.
- If the patient has a wrist-drop, place the wrist in a splint. Usually a futura splint should be available in the ED and should suffice.
- If a humeral brace is available this should be fitted along with the collar and cuff.
- There are a few absolute indications for operative fixation and under the following circumstances you should alert your senior immediately about the patient:
    - A vascular injury.
    - An open fracture.
    - An ipsilateral forearm fracture.
    - Pathological fractures, segmental fractures and fractures in the presence of poly-trauma should also be managed surgically.
    - Radial nerve palsy.
        - It is very rare for the radial nerve to be transected with these injuries. The vast majority are caused by a neuropraxia to the nerve. Patients need to be reassured as they are understandably very worried about this!
- For patients with closed isolated injuries without neurological symptoms who are ambulatory, it may be possible to discharge them home and then discuss in the morning trauma meeting.

TOP TIP

Many of these injuries can be managed successfully in a humeral brace. Once you have applied the brace and put them in a collar and cuff, a repeat x-ray after about 40 minutes is usually quite useful at getting an idea about whether the patient can be managed non-operatively. It is advisable to do this before discharging these patients from the ED as it will better inform decision-making when the x-rays are discussed at the trauma meeting.

DISTAL HUMERUS FRACTURES

BACKGROUND

Distal humerus fractures encompass a wide range of fracture types that can occur as a result of low-energy trauma, such as a fall in an elderly patient, or a high-energy injury in a younger patient.

RADIOLOGICAL ASSESSMENT

Required imaging include an AP and lateral x-rays of the entire humerus and forearm. There are typically 3 patterns of injury

1. Supra-condylar fractures.
2. Condylar fractures.
3. Complex intra-articular fractures, which usually occur in osteoporotic bone.

Make sure you look for associated injury patterns such as a dislocation at the elbow joint or a floating elbow (a distal humerus fracture with a forearm fracture).

KEY POINTS – HISTORY

In addition to the mechanism of injury, remember to ask about limb dominance and occupation as this may impact on treatment options.

It there a smoking history?

Ask about numbness/altered sensation/weakness in affected arm.

Also note the presence of significant medical co-morbidities (particularly diabetes).

EMERGENCY DEPARTMENT

KEY POINTS – CLINICAL ASSESSMENT

Exclude open wounds and assess neurovascular status.

MANAGEMENT

- Early analgesia and cast immobilisation with an above elbow backslab supported by a collar and cuff. The arm should be positioned at 90° in the cast.
- For un-displaced or minimally displaced supra-condylar or extra-articular condylar fractures there is a role for non-operative management. These patients can be brought back to a fracture clinic for review in a week.
- Displaced fractures and/or intra-articular fractures may need operative management and can either be admitted overnight, or if comfortable, sent home and contacted with an updated plan after the trauma meeting.

OLECRANON FRACTURES

BACKGROUND

Olecranon fractures usually occur as a result of low-energy injuries, such as a fall onto the elbow in an elderly patient with osteoporotic bone. Conversely, they may also occur in high-energy injuries in younger patients.

RADIOLOGICAL ASSESSMENT

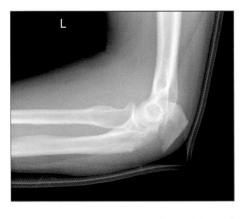

Figure 2.8. A lateral view demonstrating a displaced olecranon fracture.

It is important to get a true AP and lateral view. Inspect for the presence of an associated radial head fracture (uncommon).

EMERGENCY DEPARTMENT

KEY POINTS – HISTORY

In addition to the mechanism of injury, remember to ask about limb dominance and occupation as this may impact on treatment options.

It there a smoking history?

Ask about numbness/altered sensation/weakness in affected arm.

KEY POINTS – CLINICAL ASSESSMENT

Exclude open wounds and assess neurovascular status.

Assess active extension of the elbow BEFORE the plaster backslab is applied. Inability to do so suggests there is a discontinuity of the triceps extensor mechanism and that surgical fixation may be necessary. A good way to test this is to lie the patient's arm across a table and ask them to try to extend – this reduces the downward pull of gravity.

MANAGEMENT

- Early pain management and a broad arm sling/polysling should be given to the patient.
- The absolute indications for admission and early surgery would be:
  - An open fracture.
  - A fracture associated with a dislocated elbow.
  - A fracture associated with a neurovascular injury.
- Should any of these features be present you should inform your senior immediately.
- In the absence of the above indications, these patients can be discharged home with a view to discuss their cases at a trauma meeting within 24 hours so that they can be followed up in a clinic or timely admission for surgical management can be planned.

TOP TIPS

Look at the x-rays of the elbow thoroughly to ensure you are not missing a concomitant dislocation or Monteggia type injury pattern. Missing such injuries results in delayed management which can be harmful to the patient's clinical outcome.

EMERGENCY DEPARTMENT

ELBOW DISLOCATION

BACKGROUND

The most common type is a posterior dislocation which occurs after a fall onto a hyper-extended outstretched arm. Anterior, medial and lateral dislocations may also occur after a fall onto the arm, as well as rotational forces through the elbow joint or varus/valgus forces exerted on the elbow.

RADIOLOGICAL ASSESSMENT

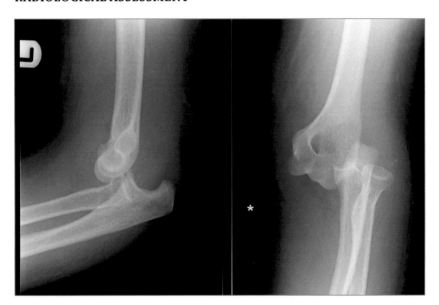

Figure 2.9. AP and lateral views demonstrating elbow dislocation.

An AP and lateral radiographic view of the elbow joint should suffice in diagnosing the dislocation and confirming the usually obvious clinical dislocation. However it is not uncommon for such injuries to be missed and patients to present to clinic several weeks later, which can have implications for recovery of function. Look carefully to see whether there are any fractures associated with the dislocation. The so-called 'terrible triad' pattern includes a posterior dislocation, a coronoid fracture and a radial head fracture. This makes the joint unstable and thus may need operative intervention.

EMERGENCY DEPARTMENT

KEY POINTS – HISTORY

Make sure you haven't missed another injury, particularly for high-energy trauma patients.

Check whether the patient is reporting any numbness, paraesthesia or weakness in the affected limb.

KEY POINTS – CLINICAL ASSESSMENT

Exclude open injuries or neurovascular compromise.

Puncture wounds can be missed especially if you are called to see the patient after the fracture has been reduced and a plaster applied by the ED team.

MANAGEMENT

- Analgesia and sedation should be administered, and the patient should be in a monitored bed (in an ED resuscitation bed) with a nurse and doctor present before any reduction is attempted. Make sure you have experience with reducing the elbow before attempting to perform a reduction without supervision.
- Assessment and documentation of the neurovascular status of the limb, pre- and post-reduction is mandatory.
- Place the patient in an above elbow backslab with a collar and cuff to support the arm. Study the post-reduction x-rays in detail to make sure the joint is reduced.
- For simple and uncomplicated dislocations that are successfully reduced, the patients should be able to go home and return to a fracture clinic in a week.
- Circumstances where you should alert your senior urgently as the patient may need immediate surgery include:
  - Failure to reduce the elbow under sedation.
  - An open fracture dislocation.
  - A dislocation with associated neurovascular injury.

> **TOP TIP**
>
> If you get called to assess a patient on the ward with increasing pain in the elbow and forearm (pre-or post-operatively) it is important to rule out a compartment syndrome. Have a low threshold for getting an urgent x-ray of the elbow to make sure that the patient has not re-dislocated.

FOREARM FRACTURES

BACKGROUND

These most commonly occur as a result of high-energy trauma such as a fall from a height or a road traffic accident. A significant number of these injuries are open fractures.

RADIOLOGICAL ASSESSMENT

AP and lateral radiographic views of the forearm are essential. Make sure that the elbow and wrist joints are also imaged. It is important to be aware of the Monteggia and Galeazzi fractures, which are less common but represent severe injuries.

EMERGENCY DEPARTMENT

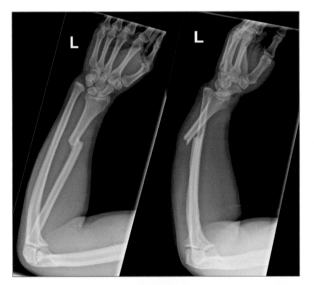

Figure 2.10. AP and lateral demonstrating a Galeazzi fracture (fracture of the distal 1/3 of the radius with a dislocation at the distal radio-ulna joint).

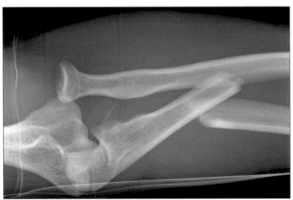

Figure 2.11 AP Radiograph demonstrating a Monteggia fracture (a fracture of the proximal 1/3 of the ulna and dislocation of the radial head).

KEY POINTS – HISTORY

In addition to the mechanism of injury, remember to ask about limb dominance and occupation as this may impact on treatment options.

It there a smoking history?

Ask about numbness/altered sensation/weakness in affected arm.

KEY POINTS – CLINICAL ASSESSMENT

Exclude open wounds and assess neurovascular status.

MANAGEMENT

- Appropriate analgesia.
- Application of an ABOVE elbow backslab is very important and will help manage the pain.
- For un-displaced or minimally displaced fractures (<50% displacement + <10 ° angulation) conservative management in a backslab for a week, followed by a full cast for a further 5 weeks is usually appropriate.
- For both bone fractures/grossly displaced/Monteggia/Galeazzi/open fractures/injuries associated with a neurovascular insult, operative treatment is necessary and such patients should be admitted. If the injuries are closed, and the forearm is very swollen, admit overnight for elevation and monitor for compartment syndrome. These should be discussed overnight with your senior.

TOP TIP

Pre- and post-operative pain is common in such patients. Open reduction and fixation of forearm fractures is a painful procedure and you may just need to adjust and improve the patient's analgesia. It is important however not to miss a compartment syndrome and you should always assess the limb for a compartment syndrome and document your assessment in the clinical notes.

EMERGENCY DEPARTMENT

DISTAL RADIUS FRACTURES

BACKGROUND

These are normally caused by a fall onto an outstretched arm. The various fracture patterns are often referred to by their eponymous names:

- Colles fracture: Low-energy, dorsally displaced, extra-articular fracture.
- Smith's fracture: Low energy, volar displaced, extra-articular fracture (reverse Colles).
- Barton's fracture: Fracture dislocation of radiocarpal joint with intra-articular fracture involving the volar or dorsal lip.

EMERGENCY
DEPARTMENT

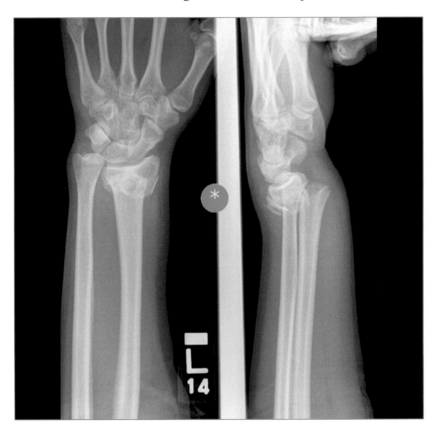

Figure 2.12. AP (a) and lateral (b) views showing a Colles fracture of the distal radius. This demonstrates the classic radiographic features: Extra-articular, dorsal displacement, shortening of the radius and radial tilt.

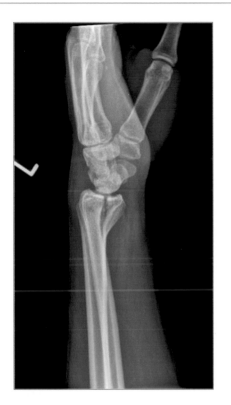

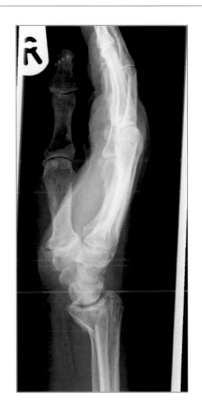

*Figure 2.13. Lateral radiograph
demonstrating Barton's fracture.
An intra-articular distal radius
fracture associated with radio-carpal
subluxation/dislocation.*

*Figure 2.14. Lateral radiograph
demonstrating a Smith's fracture.
This is an extra-articular distal
radius fracture with solar
angulation.*

RADIOLOGICAL ASSESSMENT

AP and lateral radiographic views with demonstrated an extra-articular
fracture with shortening of the radius, along with displacement and tilting.

KEY POINTS – HISTORY

In addition to the mechanism of injury, remember to ask about limb dominance and occupation as this may impact on treatment options.

It there a smoking history?

Ask about numbness/altered sensation/weakness in the hand or fingers.

KEY POINTS – CLINICAL ASSESSMENT

Exclude open wounds and assess neurovascular status.

Is there any evidence of other injuries, particularly head or spinal injury in the context of high-energy trauma?

MANAGEMENT

- If the fracture is displaced (with or without neurovascular involvement), it will need to be reduced. This is usually performed under a haematoma block (see page 113).
- Always repeat the radiograph and a neurovascular assessment post-reduction.
- As a general rule, if there is an intra-articular fracture then it requires operative management. If the reduction is inadequate, then surgery should be considered but patient co-morbidities may also sway the decision for surgery.
- Safe and ambulatory patients could go home and be contacted after discussion in the trauma meeting.
- However, if you are concerned about any neurovascular issues, then admit to the ward, elevate in a Bradford sling and reassess the patient overnight.

EMERGENCY DEPARTMENT

TOP TIPS

If the patient is in a backslab and develops numbness/paraesthesia, immediately remove the backslab and cut the underlying wool to expose the skin; do not worry about losing reduction of the fracture.

It is very common for elevation in a Bradford sling NOT to happen; make sure you insist and check it is done!

Try to avoid using eponymous names to describe the fractures unless you are SURE they are correct; sometimes best to use terms such as 'Colles-type fracture' if this occurs in a younger patient (original description was for fractures in elderly osteoporotic women). Some senior colleagues like to point this error out in meetings!

LUNATE/PERILUNATE DISLOCATION

BACKGROUND

Usually occurs after a fall onto a dorsiflexed wrist. Disruption of the carpal ligaments results in the carpus dislocating while the lunate stays in position. If the lunate dislocates and the carpus remains in place this is called a lunate dislocation.

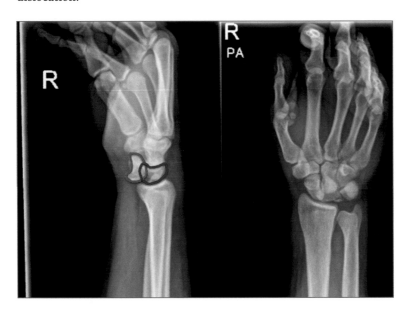

Figure 2.15. Lunate dislocation. The position of the dislocated lunate is highlighted in red. The anatomical position is highlighted in blue.

RADIOLOGICAL ASSESSMENT

Appropriate imaging and interpretation of imaging is a key part of the assessment, particularly as almost a quarter of these injuries are missed at initial presentation. Usually dislocation can be overlooked on an AP x-ray of the hand, however there are important signs to look for including a disruption in Gilula's arc and overlap of the lunate and capitate. On lateral views of the carpus and wrist joint, dislocation is often easier to see. The capitate is not aligned normally in the distal articular cup of the lunate which is best appreciated with a line drawn through the radius and lunate not intersecting the capitate.

KEY POINTS – HISTORY

In addition to the mechanism of injury, remember to ask about limb dominance and occupation as this may impact on treatment options.

It there a smoking history?

Ask about numbness/altered sensation/weakness in the hand or fingers.

KEY POINTS – CLINICAL ASSESSMENT

In almost 25% of cases, median nerve symptoms are present so it is important to perform a neurovascular assessment.

MANAGEMENT

- It is important to attempt to reduce the dislocation as soon as possible. This can be done under sedation in a monitored bed in the ED with a nurse or doctor assisting you. Traction is applied to the hand while the wrist is extended and pressure is applied onto the carpus on the palmar surface. A below elbow cast is applied with the wrist in neutral position. Following a successful reduction the hand should be elevated in a high collar and cuff and the patient should be given advice to return to hospital if pain increases or they develop signs of nerve compression in their cast.

- If closed reduction under sedation fails, patients should be admitted to have the lunate reduced as an emergency (within 6 hours) under general anaesthetic. If the closed reduction under anaesthesia fails then an open reduction should be attempted. You should inform your senior if a case like this is referred to you.
- It is highly unlikely that closed reduction forms the definitive management of these injuries. They usually require operative fixation. If a closed reduction is successfully achieved, the patient could go home, however there should be a plan in place to bring them back within a week for surgical management on an upper limb trauma list. They MUST be presented in the morning trauma meeting.
- Sometimes, an urgent referral to a dedicated regional hand unit is necessary.

TOP TIPS

These injuries are very, very easy to miss as everyone focuses on the distal radius and ulna. If you always look for the lunate whenever you assess a radiograph of the wrist, then you will be very unlikely to miss it!

EMERGENCY DEPARTMENT

BASE OF THUMB FRACTURES

BACKGROUND

Most injuries are caused by an axial force transmitted through the thumb that normally occurs after a fall on an outstretched arm. There are 3 patterns of fracture injuries affecting the base of the thumb metacarpal:

- Rolando fracture: a 3-part of T-shaped intra-articular fracture configuration.
- Bennett fracture: an intra-articular 2-part fracture.
- Extra-articular fracture.

RADIOLOGICAL ASSESSMENT

AP and lateral views radiographs of the thumb should be taken. A true AP view is commonly referred to as a Robert's view and is taken with the thumb in maximum pronation on the x-ray cassette.

KEY POINTS – HISTORY

Limb dominance, patient age and occupation are important factors to consider.

KEY POINTS – CLINICAL ASSESSMENT

The thumb is usually quite swollen and tender on palpation. If there is clinical deformity of the thumb consider a fracture-dislocation.

MANAGEMENT

- The fracture or fracture dislocation can often be reduced under local anaesthesia and sedation in the emergency room. Longitudinal traction and pronation of the thumb with pressure applied to the base of the thumb commonly reduces the fracture which should be placed in a plaster of Paris thumb spica. Repeat radiographs should be taken to check alignment before discharge.
- For fractures that fail to reduce or are intra-articular in nature, operative fixation is usually necessary. Such patients can be discharged from the ED with a view to bringing them back to the hospital for surgery within a week.

TOP TIPS

Reduction under sedation is quite difficult to achieve and hold in a plaster so do not be upset if you cannot achieve an adequate position.

BOXER'S FRACTURE (LITTLE FINGER METACARPAL NECK FRACTURE)

BACKGROUND

These fractures commonly occur after a fall onto an outstretched hand or as a result of punching. When fractures affect the neck of the metacarpal, subtle tilting of the distal fragment can cause rotational deformity of the finger and occasionally a prominent and uncomfortable palmar lump in the hand from the angulated fragment.

RADIOLOGICAL ASSESSMENT

AP, lateral and oblique view radiographs should be taken to best assess the fracture. It is important to remember when describing any metacarpal fracture (or fracture affecting the phalanges), the digit should be described as thumb, index, middle, ring or little finger. Digits should not be described as a number.

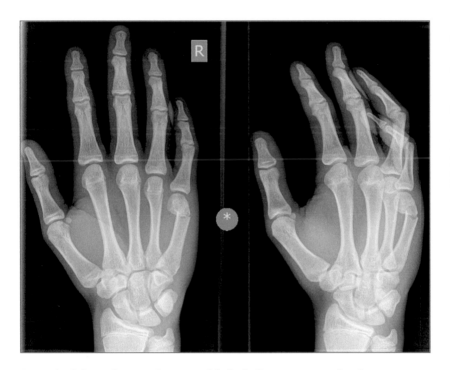

Figure 2.16. Boxer fracture. Fracture of the little finger metacarpal neck.

KEY POINTS – HISTORY

Ask about limb dominance and occupation as this may impact on treatment options.

Ask about numbness/altered sensation/weakness in the hand or fingers.

It is important to probe the mechanism of injury – often people don't report the mechanism of injury out of embarrassment especially if the injury occurred after punching someone else. These injuries can be open and a toothmark-shaped wound is seen over the knuckle. In such cases the injury is a contaminated open fracture which needs to be recognised early on.

KEY POINTS – CLINICAL ASSESSMENT

Exclude any open injuries.

Look for rotational deformity of the little finger. This is best assessed by asking the patient to make a fist and observing scissoring of the digit compared to the contralateral little finger.

MANAGEMENT

- Closed reduction in the emergency department can be attempted with a haematoma block. Traction on the metacarpal with the MCP flexed to 90° and direct pressure on the distal fragment may reduce the fracture. These injuries are normally held in an ulnar gutter plaster in an Edinburgh position (the MCP is flexed at 90° and the wrist is hyperextended).

- The majority of these are managed non-operatively but significant angulation or rotational deformities may require operative fixation. These patients can be discharged from the ED and brought back to an appropriate upper limb trauma list for surgery. The exception is in the case of open fractures where the patient should be admitted and managed as per open fracture guidelines.

TOP TIPS

Have a high index of suspicion if the history does not involve a punch. If the patient has punched someone else (or you strongly suspect this is the case) and there are scratches on the skin (i.e. an open fracture), have a low threshold to start antibiotics. The human mouth is extremely dirty and thus infection rates can be quite high. These injuries, commonly referred to as fight bite injuries, should be treated with a washout of the wound in theatre and the importance of an accurate history needs to be explained to patients who may be too embarrassed to give an accurate version of events.

LOWER LIMB

NECK OF FEMUR FRACTURES

BACKGROUND

These fractures involve the proximal femur up to 5cm below the lesser trochanter. They are usually seen after a mechanical fall in the elderly. Be particularly vigilant of the pathological fracture in osteoporotic or diseased bone. They can more rarely occur in high-energy injuries in the young, most commonly after a road traffic collision.

EMERGENCY
DEPARTMENT

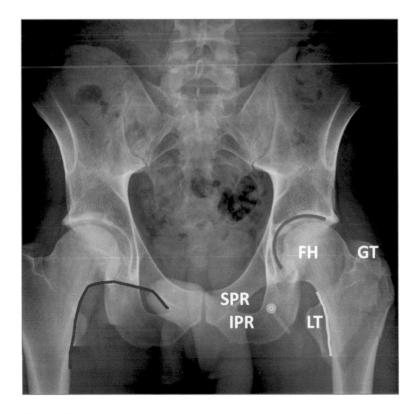

Figure 2.17. An AP pelvis radiograph demonstrating the key anatomical areas.

- *FH: Femoral head*
- *GT: Great trochanter*
- *LT: Lesser trochanter*
- *SPR: Superior pubic ramus*
- *IPR: Inferior pubic ramus*
- *Blue line: Shenton's line*
- *Yellow line: Medial calcar*
- *Red arc: Acetabulum*

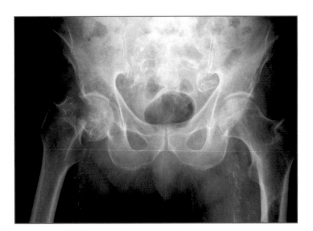

Figure 2.18. An AP pelvis view showing a right-sided intracapsular neck of femur fracture.

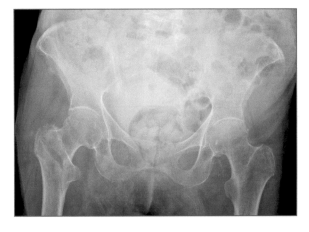

Figure 2.19. Right-sided extracapsular neck of femur fracture.

EMERGENCY DEPARTMENT

RADIOLOGICAL ASSESSMENT

Make sure that you have an AP Pelvic and lateral hip radiograph.

The most important parameter is whether the fracture is intracapsular (Figure 2.18) or extracapsular (Figure 2.19). Intracapsular fractures can be subcapital or transcervical. The distinction can be difficult depending on the rotation and quality of the radiograph.

Extracapsular fractures are either basicervical or intertrochanteric. They can also be subtrochanteric after which they become classified as proximal femoral fractures (see pages 13–14).

Comminution of the fracture is not uncommon and the fracture may made up of 2, 3 or 4 parts. Displacement of the lesser trochanter can occur.

For intracapsular fractures the Garden classification (I-IV) is commonly used to assist with treatment methods (see page 13).

KEY POINTS – HISTORY

A detailed history to illicit the mechanism of injury, medical co-morbidities and medication (esp. anticoagulants) is required, but the patient's social history will also be of vital importance to assess their rehabilitation. Therefore it is important to note the patient's:

- Age.
- Occupation (if retired what activities do they do).
- Pre-injury mobility (independent, stick, frame, wheelchair).
- Social history (who lives with them).
- Accommodation type.
- Smoking history.
- AMT Score.

KEY POINTS – CLINICAL ASSESSMENT

External rotation and shortening of the limb is a valuable sign.

Inspect for any open wounds (any evidence of an open wound requires following the open wound management protocols as per the BOA/BAPRAS guidelines).

Assess the neurovascular status of the limb, especially sciatic nerve function.

Some patients can actually weight bear if the fracture is impacted.

MANAGEMENT

- Analgesia. Consider performing a fascia iliaca local anaesthetic block.
- Most elderly patients are given IV fluids for dehydration.
- Prepare patient for surgery as invariably neck of femur fractures require surgical management.
- Blood tests (FBC, U&Es, clotting screen, group and save)
- ECG
- Urine dip stick +/- catheter with an input and output chart
- Chest x-ray: if coughing then sputum culture
- Consider oxygen administration
- Some units may require entry of data onto standardised pro-formas so check with your senior if this is required.
- If fracture difficult to delineate but high clinical suspicion present, depending on hospital availability and policy (discuss with senior) a hip CT or MRI can be performed.

EMERGENCY
DEPARTMENT

- Intracapsular fractures will require a hemiarthroplasty or a total hip replacement if they are displaced or have decreased mobility. In the active and independent fixation can be considered. Extracapsular fractures will undergo fixation using a DHS or an intramedullary nail.
- Investigate the cause of the fall: mechanical or underlying reason present.

TOP TIPS

These patients are usually elderly and can deteriorate rapidly after admission, and therefore regular review overnight is required.

If oral analgesia was not adequate consider IV or ask the anesthetist to perform a fascia iliaca block.

Contact the family of the patient or speak to their carer to get a collateral history.

FEMORAL SHAFT FRACTURES

BACKGROUND

This is a high-energy traumatic injury frequently associated with life-threatening conditions, often as a result of RTC or a fall from a height. Low-energy femoral fractures should raise the suspicion of a pathological fracture especially in the elderly.

RADIOLOGICAL ASSESSMENT

Make sure that you obtain an AP pelvic x-ray, along with an AP and a lateral x-ray of the whole femur and an AP and lateral of both the ipsilateral hip and ipsilateral knee. If there is suspicion of a pathological fracture then discussion with a senior and obtaining a CT scan would be indicated.

KEY POINTS – HISTORY

The focus again should be on the details of the injury, medical co-morbidities and social history.

KEY POINTS – CLINICAL ASSESSMENT

Initial evaluation of these patients should be along the ATLS protocol.

Exclude open injuries and neurovascular compromise.

The thigh can be tense, swollen and short. If a period of time has passed, bruising might start to appear, more commonly in the posterior aspect where blood is pooling (up to 1.5L blood loss can occur).

Assess neurovascular status of the limb, especially the function of the branches of the sciatic nerve (tibial and common peroneal nerve) as they usually divide around the popliteal region.

MANAGEMENT

- ATLS protocol should be instigated with the trauma team present in a high-energy mechanism of injury.
- Analgesia – think about asking the radiology or ED team to consider performing a fascia iliaca local anaesthetic block.
- Investigate the cause of the fall and the energy involved: mechanical or underlying reason (pathological).
- Full secondary survey needs to be completed and documented.
- Monitor patient overnight for pain management and risk of compartment syndrome.
- Surgical treatment would include either an antegrade intramedullary nail, retrograde intramedullary nail, external fixator (in poly-trauma or open wound) or ORIF – depending on the fracture configuration and proximity or involvement of the joint.

EMERGENCY DEPARTMENT

TOP TIPS

When these injuries occur in the elderly population, they should be treated just like NOF fracture patients (see previous topic).

If oral analgesia was not adequate consider IV or ask the anesthetist to perform a fascia iliaca block and/or in-line skin traction of 5lb or Thomas splint.

Always look for a neck of femur fracture when you see a femoral shaft fracture, and ensure an x-ray of the hip is obtained.

HIP DISLOCATION

BACKGROUND

A native hip dislocation is a rare injury. It occurs with high-energy trauma from an RTC (dashboard injury) or fall from a height. Due to the high energy involved, there is a high incidence of associated injuries. A dislocation following a total hip replacement or a hip hemiarthroplasty is more common than a native hip dislocation.

RADIOLOGICAL ASSESSMENT

An AP and lateral radiograph of the pelvis is usually requested to confirm the clinically apparent dislocation and to also exclude any fractures. 90% of dislocations are posterior while 10% are anterior.

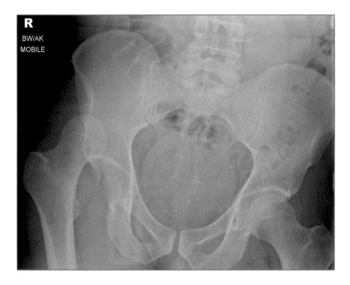

Figure 2.20. A native right hip dislocation seen on AP radiograph.

Look carefully for fractures of the femoral neck, head and acetabulum; if any doubt then a CT may be needed to exclude these fractures.

KEY POINTS – HISTORY

The focus again should be on the details of the injury, medical co-morbidities and social history. Ask about numbness in the foot (looking for sciatic nerve injury).

KEY POINTS – CLINICAL ASSESSMENT

Inspect for any open wounds (any evidence of an open wound requires following the open wound management protocols as per the BOA/BAPRAS guidelines).

Assess vascularity: femoral, popliteal, tibialis anterior and posterior and dorsalis pedis pulses.

Full detailed neurological assessment needs to be documented. Sciatic nerve injuries and entrapment of the nerve following reduction can occur.

The position of the leg will indicate the direction of the dislocation: if the leg is internally rotated and adducted then it's a posterior dislocation (90%), and if it's abducted and externally rotated it's an anterior dislocation (10%).

MANAGEMENT

- ATLS protocol should be instigated with the trauma team present in a high-energy mechanism of injury. 95% of dislocations have associated injuries.
- Please give adequate analgesia. The best analgesia in this case will be relocating the hip. A neurovascular examination **MUST** be performed and documented **PRIOR** to any intervention (10–20% sciatic nerve injury).
- A closed reduction under sedation in the ED should be attempted followed by a full GA with paralysis in theatre if the initial attempts are unsuccessful. This should be performed ASAP and within 6 hours. This is contraindicated in the presence of the femoral neck fracture.
- Full secondary survey needs to be completed and documented.
- A neurovascular examination **MUST** be performed and documented **AFTER** reduction of the hip. The sciatic nerve can get trapped with the joint during reduction; this would require urgent surgical exploration.
- If reduction is not achieved immediately in the ED, consider skin traction with 5lb over the end of the bed for comfort. Re-check the neurovascular status following application of traction/splint.

EMERGENCY DEPARTMENT

TOP TIPS

Native hip dislocations are an orthopaedic emergency and need to be reduced as soon as possible. Dislocations involving a prosthesis (e.g. in the presence of a total hip replacement) can wait until the morning, provided there is no evidence of neurovascular impairment. Alert your senior if such a case comes in during your shift.

DISTAL FEMORAL FRACTURES

BACKGROUND

This is a high-energy traumatic injury in the young patient often as a result of an RTC or a fall from a height. Low energy distal femoral fractures should raise the suspicion of a pathological fracture but these can be seen in the osteoporotic elderly population.

RADIOLOGICAL ASSESSMENT

Make sure that you obtain an AP radiograph of the pelvis as well as an AP and a lateral radiograph of the entire femur and knee joint – to ensure no other injury is missed. It is key to appreciate that a fracture of the distal femur may have an undisplaced intra-articular extension. If suspicion is present then discuss with a senior as a CT scan may be warranted.

KEY POINTS – HISTORY

The focus again should be on the details of the injury, medical co-morbidities and social history.

KEY POINTS – CLINICAL ASSESSMENT

Initial evaluation of these patients should be along the ATLS protocol.

Thigh can be tense and swollen; monitor for compartment syndrome.

Inspect for any open wounds (any evidence of an open wound requires following the open wound management protocols as per BOAST guidelines (see page 86)).

Assess neurovascular status of the limb, especially the function of the branches of the sciatic nerve (tibial and common peroneal nerve) as they usually divide around the popliteal region.

EMERGENCY DEPARTMENT

Palpate distal pulses and CRT. There is an increased incidence of popliteal artery injury in displaced fractures. If pulse is not present alert the Vascular/Plastic Surgeons and discuss with your radiologist to obtain an urgent CT angiogram.

MANAGEMENT

- ATLS protocol should be instigated with the trauma team present due to the high-energy mechanism.
- Analgesia.
- Once examination performed and documented, apply an above knee POP to include the ankle for preliminary stability and pain relief.
- Investigate the cause of the fall and the energy involved: mechanical or underlying reason (pathological).
- Full secondary survey needs to be completed and documented.
- Ensure the POP applied is comfortable and does not put excessive pressure on any of the vulnerable bony areas or at the back of the thigh. Repeat the neurovascular examination and document it following POP application.
- Monitor patient overnight for pain management and risk of compartment syndrome.
- Non-operative treatment is rare and reserved for unwell patients with multiple co-morbidities, non-ambulant patients or undisplaced fractures. In this situation this fracture can be treated initially with a POP followed by a hinged knee brace. Surgical treatment would include either a retrograde intramedullary nail, an external fixator (in poly-trauma or open injuries) or with an open reduction and internal fixation.

EMERGENCY DEPARTMENT

TOP TIPS

If oral analgesia was not adequate consider IV analgesia or ask the anaesthetist to perform a block and/or skin traction of 5lb. Usually the POP improves pain symptoms.

Monitor for compartment syndrome before and after patient has definitive treatment.

Internal compartmental blood can be significant (1.5L within an adult thigh) and haemodynamic instability in the form of shock can be a delayed response.

TIBIAL PLATEAU FRACTURES

BACKGROUND

Tibial plateau fractures are periarticular fractures of the proximal tibia and are often associated with soft tissue knee injuries, and occasionally neurovascular injuries.

RADIOLOGICAL ASSESSMENT

AP and lateral x-ray of the knee with consideration of an AP and lateral of the tibia if distal extension is present. A lipohaemarthrosis (horizontal line within the suprapatella region of the knee on a lateral radiograph) is an indication of an occult intra-articular injury. This represents a separation between the blood due to the injury and the bone marrow fat that has escaped from the fracture site.

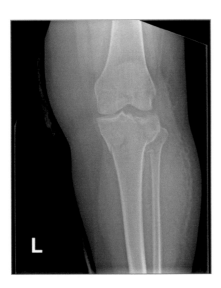

Figure 2.21. AP radiograph showing a tibial plateau fracture; both medial and lateral aspects (Schatzker V, see common classification of fractures chapter, page 14).

Note that the lateral tibial plateau is convex in shape while medial is concave.

An articular step of over 5mm is usually considered significant.

Most of these injuries requiring surgical intervention need a CT scan for operative planning.

The Schatzker classification is the one that is most used in this injury.

EMERGENCY DEPARTMENT

KEY POINTS – HISTORY

The focus again should be on the details of the injury, medical co-morbidities and social history.

KEY POINTS – CLINICAL ASSESSMENT

Initial evaluation of these patients should be along the ATLS protocol.

Knee swelling and a tense painful effusion is common.

Palpate distal pulses and CRT. There is an increased incidence of popliteal artery injury in displaced plateau fractures at the level of the trifurcation. Type IV (medial plateau) is also considered part of the spectrum of knee dislocation and one should have a high index of suspicion for a neurovascular injury. If the pulse is weak in comparison or not present alert the Vascular/Plastic Surgeons, perform an ankle-brachial index measurement and discuss with your radiologist to obtain an urgent CT angiogram. Popliteal artery injury could be in the form of an intimal tear that is detected radiologically.

Assess neurovascular status of the limb, especially the function of the branches of the sciatic nerve (tibial and common peroneal nerve) as they usually divide around the popliteal region. The common peroneal nerve can be compressed secondary to swelling around the lateral aspect of the knee.

EMERGENCY DEPARTMENT

MANAGEMENT

- ATLS protocol should be instigated with the trauma team present due to the high-energy mechanism.
- Once examination performed and documented, apply an above knee POP to include the ankle for preliminary stability and pain relief.
- If a knee dislocation is suspected, alert your senior.
- Investigate the cause of the fall and the energy involved: mechanical or underlying reason (pathological).
- Full secondary survey needs to be completed and documented.
- Ensure the POP applied is comfortable and does not put excessive pressure to any of the vulnerable bony areas or at the back of the thigh. Repeat the neurovascular examination and document it following POP application.
- Non-operative treatment is reserved for the non-ambulatory elderly +/- co-morbidities and the undisplaced lateral plateau fracture. Surgical treatment would include a temporizing spanning external

fixator for the soft tissues to settle prior to surgery. This process can be 2 weeks. Most of these fractures are treated with ORIF using anatomical or juxta-articular plates, but with severely comminuted fractures a circular frame may be advised.

TOP TIPS

Associated soft tissue injuries include meniscal tears, ACL injury and collateral ligament injuries. An MRI is useful to assess soft tissue injuries.

KNEE DISLOCATION

BACKGROUND

This devastating injury can be caused by low or high energy trauma. High energy is usually from an RTC (dashboard injury) while low energy are usually sport injuries and also associated with morbid obesity. This injury leads to significant soft tissue injury. Importantly, it can be associated with both nerve and vascular injuries.

RADIOLOGICAL ASSESSMENT

AP and lateral radiographs of the affected knee should be obtained, however it is clinically very obvious when the joint is dislocated. You should NOT delay reduction of the joint to obtain the radiographs.

Note that the radiographs could be normal if spontaneous reduction has occurred or has been reduced by the emergency staff. This does not mean the knee is normal!

Look for asymmetry or difference in joint space.

If you do have a radiograph of the joint dislocated, it can be described based on the displacement of the tibia (Anterior > Posterior > Lateral > Medial > Rotational.)

KEY POINTS – HISTORY

The focus again should be on the details of the injury, medical co-morbidities and social history.

KEY POINTS – CLINICAL ASSESSMENT

Inspect for any open wounds (any evidence of an open wound requires following the open wound management protocols as per the BOA/BAPRAS guidelines).

Assess vascularity both palpation and CRT: popliteal, tibialis anterior and posterior and dorsalis pedis pulses (can be as high as 50% if intimal tears are included).

Full detailed neurological assessment needs to be documented. Common peroneal nerve injuries 25% and tibial less common)

Position of the leg will indicate the direction of the dislocation: if the leg is internally rotated and adducted then it's a posterior dislocation, and if it's abducted and externally rotated it's an anterior dislocation.

MANAGEMENT

- ATLS protocol should be instigated with the trauma team present in a high-energy mechanism of injury.
- Analgesia (optimise oral analgesia as per the analgesic). The best analgesia is reduction of the knee. Place in an above knee backslab once reduced.
- Neurovascular examination should be performed prior to any intervention.
- Relocation in the ED should be considered and should be performed without delay in the pulseless foot. Anaesthetic input would be beneficial for adequate sedation.
- If no deformity is present then the knee could have spontaneously reduced. Other signs include: swelling, effusion, bruising, abrasions.
- There is an increased incidence of popliteal artery injury. If pulse is weak in comparison to the other limb, or not present, alert the Vascular/Plastic Surgeons, perform an ankle-brachial pressure index (ABPI) and discuss with your radiologist to obtain an urgent CT angiogram. Popliteal artery injury could be in the form of an intimal tear that is detected radiologically. If pulses are absent following reduction, immediate exploration is warranted.
- Assess the function of the tibial and common peroneal nerve. They can be compressed by the swelling or the dislocation and documentation and monitoring is key.

EMERGENCY DEPARTMENT

- Stability is sometimes difficult to assess in an acute injury, but if tolerated should be performed.
- Full secondary survey needs to be completed and documented.
- An MRI scan should be obtained following reduction to assess the extent of the soft tissue injury. This will guide further management.

TOP TIPS

This injury is under-diagnosed as 50% spontaneously reduce before arrival. Do not dismiss a confident history.

TIBIAL SHAFT FRACTURES

BACKGROUND

A tibial shaft fracture is the most common long bone fracture. It may occur either as a direct blow or as a result of a twisting (torsion) injury. There is a high incidence of associated open fractures due to the reduced soft tissue envelope in the leg.

RADIOLOGICAL ASSESSMENT

An AP and lateral radiograph of the tibia, with consideration of an AP and lateral of the knee (tibial plateau) or ankle (tibial plafond) if the fracture is close to either joint, should be obtained. The presence of a lipohaemarthrosis is an indication of an occult intra-articular injury.

KEY POINTS – HISTORY

The focus again should be on the details of the injury, medical co-morbidities and social history.

KEY POINTS – CLINICAL ASSESSMENT

Exclude neurovascular compromise and open injuries.

If pulse is weak in comparison or not present alert the Vascular/Plastic Surgeons, perform an ankle-brachial index measurement and discuss with your radiologist to obtain an urgent CT angiogram. Popliteal artery injury could be in the form of an intimal tear that is detected radiologically. Full neurological assessment needs to be documented. This is to include the superficial and deep peroneal nerves, the sural nerve, the saphenous nerve, tibial nerve. Numbness, paresthesia or weakness should raise the suspicion of a nerve injury.

MANAGEMENT

- ATLS protocol should be instigated with the trauma team present in a high-energy mechanism of injury.
- Analgesia
- Once examination performed and documented, apply an above knee backslab to include the ankle for preliminary stability and pain relief.
- Full secondary survey needs to be completed and documented.
- Ensure the POP applied is comfortable and does not put excessive pressure on any of the vulnerable bony areas or at the back of the thigh. Repeat the neurovascular examination and document it following POP application.
- Monitor patient overnight for pain management and risk of compartment syndrome. The risk is **HIGHER** in closed tibial fractures.
- Non-operative treatment is reserved for the non-ambulatory elderly +/- co-morbidities and the undisplaced fractures. In this situation this fracture can be treated initially with a POP and elevation and non-weight bearing.
- Surgical treatment includes the application of an external fixator in open fractures until definitive treatment is deemed appropriate. Most of these fractures are treated with an antegrade (infra- or supra-patellar) intramedullary nail.

EMERGENCY DEPARTMENT

TOP TIPS

Elevation and icing is key. If pain is severe and unremitting think of compartment syndrome by removing the plaster and assessing the limb clinically. **DO NOT WORRY** about the fracture displacing, this is easily corrected, but a missed compartment syndrome is disastrous.

TIBIAL PLAFOND FRACTURES

BACKGROUND

Also known as a 'pilon fracture', it is usually associated with a high-energy load injury with significant surrounding soft tissue trauma. It most commonly arises from a road traffic accident or a fall from a height.

RADIOLOGICAL ASSESSMENT

AP, lateral and mortise radiograph of the ankle and a full length tibia/fibula radiograph to reveal any fracture extension.

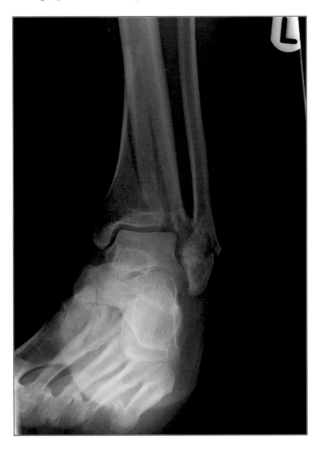

Figure 2.22. Tibial plafond (Pilon) fracture.

KEY POINTS – HISTORY

The focus again should be on the details of the injury, medical co-morbidities and social history.

KEY POINTS – CLINICAL ASSESSMENT

Full neurological assessment needs to be documented. This is to include the superficial and deep peroneal nerves, the sural nerve, the saphenous nerve, tibial nerve. Numbness, paresthesia or weakness should raise the suspicion of a nerve injury.

Exclude open fractures.

MANAGEMENT

- Analgesia.
- Once examination performed and documented, correct obvious deformity if present under adequate analgesia and apply a below knee POP for preliminary stability and pain relief.
- Full secondary survey needs to be completed and documented, especially any associated knee, hip/pelvis & spine injuries because of axial loading of the tibia caused by the injury.
- Ensure the POP applied is comfortable and does not put excessive pressure on any of the vulnerable bony areas. Repeat the neurovascular examination and document it following POP application.
- Monitor patient overnight for pain management and risk of compartment syndrome.
- Non-operative treatment is reserved for the non-ambulatory elderly +/- co-morbidities and the undisplaced fractures.
- Surgical treatment includes an external fixator in open fractures or significant soft tissue trauma until definitive treatment is deemed appropriate.

TOP TIPS

Fracture blisters are not uncommon and thus the skin condition needs to be monitored.

EMERGENCY DEPARTMENT

ANKLE FRACTURES

BACKGROUND

Most are simple twisting injuries such as stepping off a kerb.

RADIOLOGICAL ASSESSMENT

AP, lateral and mortise (15-20° of internal rotation of the leg so that
the x-ray beam is perpendicular to the inter-malleolar line) radiographs of
the ankle.

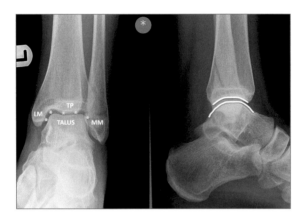

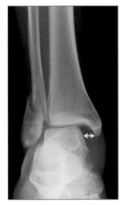

Figure 2.23. Anatomy of the ankle.

- *LM: Lateral malleolus*
- *MM: Medial malleolus*
- *TP: Tibial plafond*
- *Medial clear space: the distance between the tibial plafond and*

the articular surface of the talus should be the same throughout the joint (yellow stars)

- *Congruency between TP and talus on lateral radiograph*

Figure 2.24. Weber B fracture of the lateral malleolus with evidence of talar shift (widening of the medial clear space).

Look for evidence of dislocation of subluxation of the ankle joint. This can be
seen on the AP/mortise view as widening of the medial clear space (between
the medial malleolus and the medial aspect of the talus) or talar shift (where
the tibial plafond and articular surface of the talus are no longer parallel to
each other) and on the lateral view where the talus is not seated congruently
underneath the tibial plafond.

Lateral malleolus fractures can be classified using the Weber Classification
system (see page 15).

KEY POINTS – HISTORY

The focus again should be on the details of the injury, medical co-morbidities and social history.

KEY POINTS – CLINICAL ASSESSMENT

Exclude open injuries and neurovascular compromise

MANAGEMENT

- Analgesia.
- Once neurovascular examination is performed and documented, correct obvious deformity if present under adequate analgesia, and apply a below knee POP backslab for preliminary stability and pain relief.
- If there is evidence of a fracture dislocation/subluxation, this is best reduced in the ED and then placed into a plaster. This is usually done by the ED team so ask them for assistance; it is more than a one person job!
- You must get another radiograph in plaster to ensure the fracture is in an acceptable position.
- Full secondary survey needs to be completed and documented.
- Management depends on the stability of the ankle and fracture displacement. Many can be treated in plaster or with a walking boot if the configuration is stable. Others require surgical intervention usually in the form of ORIF and screws to the medial malleolus if fractured.
- Very unstable fractures with excessive soft tissue swelling may require an external fixator prior to definitive treatment. It is relatively common to have to wait around 5–10 days for swelling to come down prior to having an operation.

EMERGENCY DEPARTMENT

TOP TIPS

Elevation and icing is key. The leg should be elevated ABOVE the level of the heart to help reduce the swelling.

TARSOMETATARSAL FRACTURE-DISLOCATION

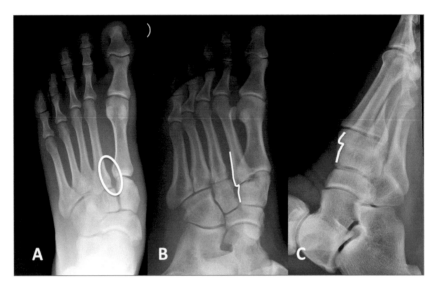

Figure 2.25.

A: AP radiograph

- *Disruption of the line along the medial base of the second metatarsal and the medial edge of the middle cuneiform*
- *Widening of the interval between the first and second metatarsal bases*
- *Sometimes a small bony fragment from the base of the 2ⁿᵈ metatarsal can be seen (within the circled area). This represents an avulsion of the Lisfranc ligament and is called the 'fleck sign'.*

B: Oblique radiograph

- *Malalignment of base of the fourth metatarsal and the cuboid*
- *Disruption of the line along the medial base of the second metatarsal and the medial edge of the middle cuneiform*

C: Lateral radiograph

- *Dorsal displacement/ subluxation of the proximal base of the first or second metatarsal*

BACKGROUND

This is a rare injury and is eponymously recognized as a 'Lisfranc fracture'. The Lisfranc joint complex consists of three articulations which include the tarsometatarsal joint, intermetatarsal joint, intertarsal joint. The Lisfranc ligament is critical in the stability of the second metatarsal and the maintenance of the midfoot arch. It is an interosseous ligament spanning the medial cuneiform to the base of 2nd metatarsal on the plantar surface. This ligament tightens when the foot is abducted and pronated.

It is usually a high-energy injury caused by an indirect rotational force and axial load through a hyper plantar flexed foot. While usually caused through a road traffic accident or a fall from a height, it can also be secondary to twisting in sporting injuries which causes a disruption in the tarsometatarsal joint.

RADIOLOGICAL ASSESSMENT

AP, lateral and oblique radiograph of the foot as well as a comparison with stress weight-bearing AP (especially if a purely ligamentous injury).

KEY POINTS – HISTORY

The focus again should be on the details of the injury, medical co-morbidities and social history.

KEY POINTS – CLINICAL ASSESSMENT

Swelling and pain present around the foot, usually associated with significant foot swelling around the midfoot.

Inspect for any open wounds.

Assess vascularity of the foot (palpation of the distal pulses might be difficult if excessive swelling is present, but CRT should not be compromised).

Medial plantar bruising (on the sole of the foot) is commonly seen with this injury.

EMERGENCY DEPARTMENT

MANAGEMENT

- Analgesia.
- No splints are necessary, elevation and icing is key, and should be a priority.
- Monitor for compartment syndrome in moderate/severe cases; this may require admission for 24 hours.
- A CT might be required to exclude this injury if radiographs are unremarkable.

TOP TIPS

This is an uncommon injury that is commonly missed. If you see a patient with a very swollen foot but you cannot see anything obviously fractured, admit overnight for observation. They can have further imaging the next day after a senior review if deemed necessary.

METATARSAL FRACTURES

BACKGROUND

This is one of the most common injuries of the foot, the 5th metatarsal (MT) being most common. The 2nd MT however is the longest and most commonly involved in stress fractures due to repetitive microtrauma e.g. marching soldiers.

The mechanism is either a direct crush injury which tends to be associated with significant soft tissue injury, indirect twisting of the forefoot onto the hindfoot (most common) or stress fractures. Stress fractures of the 2nd MT are called March fractures, while those at the base of the 5th MT are called Jones fractures.

RADIOLOGICAL ASSESSMENT

AP, lateral and oblique radiographs of the foot should be obtained.

Review alignment of metatarsals looking at the location of the fracture, the type of fracture (transverse, oblique, spiral), the amount of displacement and angulation and any evidence of articular involvement.

KEY POINTS – HISTORY

The focus again should be on the details of the injury, medical co-morbidities and social history.

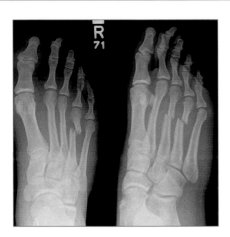

Figure 2.26. AP and oblique radiographs of the foot showing complete oblique fractures through the third and fourth metatarsals and an incomplete fracture through the second metatarsal.

KEY POINTS – CLINICAL ASSESSMENT

Swelling and pain present around the foot, usually associated with foot swelling and inability to bear weight.

Inspect for any open wounds (any evidence of an open wound requires following the open wound management protocols as per the BOA/BAPRAS guidelines).

Assess vascularity of the foot (distal pulses and CRT) and neurology around the foot and toe in question.

Bruising is common.

MANAGEMENT

- Analgesia.
- No splints are necessary initially; elevation and icing is key. However if the patient is in pain, they can have a below knee backslab applied.
- Mostly treated with a stiff insole or a boot weight bearing as tolerated. More caution and follow up required for displaced base of the 5th metatarsal fracture due to risk of non-union due to the pull of peroneus brevis.

TOP TIPS

If severe swelling is present review the midfoot and consider a Lisfranc injury or compartment syndrome, especially when multiple metatarsal fractures are present. Admit and elevate the patient overnight if the swelling and pain is significant.

PAEDIATRIC INJURIES

Dealing with paediatric patients tends to cause a bit more anxiety than adult patients. This is probably due to a number of reasons:

- A younger patient may not be able to communicate with you directly or in much detail.
- A child may be uncooperative.
- Difficult radiographs to interpret due to the presence of growth plates.
- Having to deal with parents/relatives.

The key is to stay calm and approach the paediatric patient in the exact same way that you would any other patient. Try to appear relaxed and smile! The patient will be frightened being in hospital and your body language can help calm them down. It will also appear to the parents that you are in control and comfortable.

Other tips include

- Try to interact with the child.
- Offer to examine the child whilst they sit on their parent's lap.
- Examine the uninjured limb/parent/cuddly toy first to show the child what you intend to do.

DISTAL FOREARM FRACTURES

BACKGROUND

There is usually a history of trauma and the child or parent/guardian may be able to tell you the history or localize to the affected region. It is important to be aware of the variety of eponymous names that are associated with these injuries as many are used interchangeably and often imprecisely.

Extra-articular fractures include:

- *Buckle (Torus) fracture*: this is a 'compression' of the bone that is characterised by bulging of the cortex with no visible fracture lines.
- *Greenstick fracture:* bend in the cortex on one side and a visible fracture in the bone cortex on the other side. The fracture is usually incomplete.

EPIPHYSEAL FRACTURES

These are fractures that involve the epiphyseal plate or growth plate of a bone. These are important as they can result in premature closure and therefore limb shortening and abnormal growth. They are most commonly described via the Salter-Harris classification (see page 16).

RADIOLOGICAL ASSESSMENT

Generally plain radiographs in at least 2 planes of the affected region should be obtained (e.g. an AP and a lateral). Sometimes you must also include the joint above and below; this is usually done after clinical evaluation.

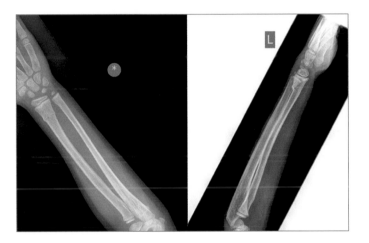

Figure 2.27. Buckle or Torus fracture of the distal radius.

KEY POINTS – HISTORY

Is there a history of trauma/falls?

How long has the child been complaining of pain?

Have they been reluctant to use that particular limb?

KEY POINTS – CLINICAL ASSESSMENT

Note any visible deformities and identify any swelling around or effusion within the surrounding joints.

MANAGEMENT

- Assess the neurovascular structure of the limb.
    - If the child is too young or too distressed to follow commands, check for distal pulses and whether they are moving the digits.
    - If there is any concern, alert your senior IMMEDIATELY.
- Look for any obvious deformity.
    - In cases of severe deformity, urgent manipulation, usually under sedation or general anaesthesia should be consider. Alert your senior IMMEDIATELY.

- If there is no obvious/subtle deformity and the limb is neurovascularly intact, then a backslab should be applied.
  - The limb should be re-imaged with radiographs.
  - The limb should be reassessed post plaster for neurovascular integrity.
- There is quite a wide acceptable angle of deformity that can be accepted in children as their bones tend to remodel.
- If you feel the fracture needs a surgical intervention, then the patient should be admitted and the limb elevated to reduce the swelling.
- If you feel the fracture can be managed conservatively, then the patient can be discharged home but take a contact number so that they can be called after discussion in the trauma meeting.

TOP TIPS

If the child is very distressed/uncooperative, then ask the parent/guardian to assess the pulse and sensation in the affected limb under your guidance.

SUPRACONDYLAR ELBOW FRACTURES

BACKGROUND

This is often caused by a fall onto an outstretched arm. An extension type of displacement is by far more common than the flexion type (95% vs 5% respectively).

RADIOLOGICAL ASSESSMENT

Several radiological lines should be known in order to avoid missing subtle fractures (see Figure 2.28)

KEY POINTS – HISTORY

As with all injuries, the mechanism of trauma is important.

Ask about the presence of numbness or tingling.

When did the child last eat or drink (especially important in cases of displaced fractures).

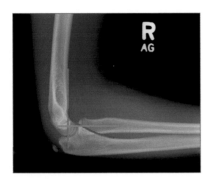

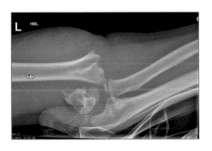

Figure 2.28. Anatomy of the elbow.

- *Anterior coronoid line (red): a line drawn along the coronoid fossa of the proximal ulna; it should just touch the capitellum anteriorly*
- *Anterior humeral line (blue): a line drawn down the anterior cortex of the humerus should transect the middle third of the capitellum on a lateral radiograph*
- *Radiocapitellar line (green): a line drawn down the radial neck should intersect the capitellum*

Figure 2.29. A Gartland III displaced supracondylar fracture (see page 16).

KEY POINTS – CLINICAL ASSESSMENT

Perform detailed neurology assessment of the median, ulna and radial nerve.

Assess for presence of radial and ulna pulse at the level of the wrist.

Assess the warmth of the hand.

Assess the capillary refill time.

MANAGEMENT

- In the case of Gartland I fractures, these can be managed in either a backslab (for comfort) or even a simple polysling.
- Generally grade II and III types tend to undergo operative fixation. In cases of grade III, the elbow can swell quite dramatically overnight and thus many surgeons tend to operate as soon as possible.

TOP TIPS

ALWAYS alert your senior if you see a displaced supracondylar fracture in a child.

CLAVICLE FRACTURES

BACKGROUND

Fractures involving the clavicle are the most common childhood fractures and are caused by a fall onto the shoulder.

RADIOLOGICAL ASSESSMENT

Usually an AP and a 45 degree cephalic view are requested.

KEY POINTS – HISTORY

As with all injuries, the mechanism of trauma is important.

Ask about the presence of numbness or tingling.

KEY POINTS – CLINICAL ASSESSMENT

Look for localised tenderness over the fracture site, with a palpable 'bump'.

Assess the skin for signs of compromise over the fracture site.

Perform a neurological assessment of the median, ulna and radial nerve.

IMMEDIATE MANAGEMENT
- Analgesia.
- Broad arm sling.
- Generally closed fractures are managed non-operatively, even if there is a moderate degree of displacement as remodelling occurs.

LIMPING CHILD

This is quite a common presenting complaint to any ED. It can be very difficult to obtain an accurate history because either the child is too young to communicate directly with you, or they are frightened and thus not cooperative. In such cases, it is important to liaise with the parent/guardian of the child and get as much information about the problem as possible.

Generally, you need to be thinking of several diagnoses and use clinical, radiological and biochemical parameters to exclude

1. Fracture/Trauma
2. Septic Joint

3. Slipped Upper Femoral Epiphysis (SUFE).

4. Transient Synovitis (diagnosis of exclusion).

GENERAL INVESTIGATIONS *(USUALLY REQUESTED BY ED PRIOR TO REFERRAL)*

1. Appropriate radiographs of the affected bone/joint in 2 views.

2. Biochemical markers – specifically white cell count (WCC) and inflammatory markers (CRP and/or ESR).

The typical fractures have already been discussed, but the septic joint in a child, SUFE and transient synovitis and in particular their management in the acute setting are outlined in more detail below:

SEPTIC JOINT

BACKGROUND

Usually there is no history of trauma but the parent/guardian may mention that the child is either limping or not fully using the affected limb.

RADIOLOGICAL ASSESSMENT

Generally, plain radiographs do not add anything to the diagnosis however should be requested as a means of excluding other pathology within the differential diagnosis process.

KEY POINTS – HISTORY

How long has the child been complaining of a painful joint?

Are they limping? If so for how long?

Have they been pyrexial at any time?

Is there any current or recent illness?

KEY POINTS – CLINICAL ASSESSMENT

Is the child febrile? But, be cautious in an afebrile child with clinical symptoms as they may have had prior antipyrexial agents which may mask a true pyrexia.

Are the affected joints swollen? If so are they erythematous or warm to touch compared to the contralateral side?

EMERGENCY DEPARTMENT

Ask the child to mobilise or make use of the affected limb.

Is passive examination painful?

Observe how the child holds the limb at rest

- In cases of septic joints, the position of flexion tends to stretch the joint capsule less and thus be more comfortable.

You may find it useful to consider the findings in terms of the Kocher Criteria, where a point is given for each of the following:

> Non-weight bearing of the affected side
>
> ESR > 40
>
> Fever > 38.5°C
>
> White Cell Count (WCC) > 12,000

A score of 1 represents a 3% likelihood of septic arthritis, 2 represents a 40% likelihood and 3 or 4 represent a 93% or 99% likelihood respectively.

MANAGEMENT

- If the child is profoundly septic, alert your senior IMMEDIATELY.
- If the child is relatively well and stable haemodynamically, then they should be admitted for further investigations. Most departments tend to have a set protocol for investigating a paediatric septic joint; this usually involves an ultrasound to look for a joint effusion.

TOP TIPS

Always inform the paediatric team of admissions for a potential septic joint as they will also review the child and exclude any other potential cause of sepsis.

SLIPPED UPPER (CAPITAL) FEMORAL EPIPHYSIS

BACKGROUND

There may be a history of trauma however it can sometimes be of insidious onset, for example of low-energy fall. This injury is essential is a fracture across the growth plate. As a result, the femoral head stays in its normal position within the acetabulum but the femur and the femoral neck displaces anteriorly. The aim of treatment is to stop further displacement (so called 'slippage'). In case of large, neglected slips, impingement of the hip, avascular necrosis of the femoral head, chondrolysis, degenerative osteoarthritis and proximal femoral deformity and leg length discrepancy can occur.

RADIOLOGICAL ASSESSMENT

An AP (Figure 2.30) and frog leg lateral (Figure 2.31) of the pelvis should be requested.

KEY POINTS – HISTORY

The age of child is commonly 12–14 years.

Is there a history of trauma/falls?

How long has the child been complaining of pain?

Have they been reluctant to use that particular limb?

- Assess for the presence of knee pain and this may be the only clue!

Past medical history

- Associated with hypothyroidism, osteodystrophy and growth hormone treatment.

KEY POINTS – CLINICAL ASSESSMENT

More common in obese children

Any visible deformities?

Any effusions around the surrounding joints?

Assess active/passive range of hip motion. Compare it to the contralateral side.

MANAGEMENT

- Based on the degree of slippage and the chronicity of the presentation, surgical intervention is sometimes necessary.
- All patients with this condition MUST be admitted for more senior review and discussion of treatment options.
- In around 15% of cases, the abnormality may be bilateral and require surgical intervention. Counselling of the child and their parents/guardians is mandatory.

TOP TIPS

Beware the child complaining of knee pain. Always examine the hip joint above and request appropriate radiographs if necessary!

EMERGENCY DEPARTMENT

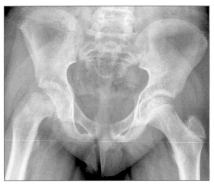

Figure 2.30.

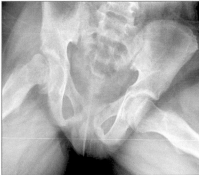

Figure 2.31.

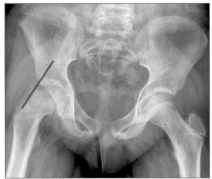

Figure 2.32.

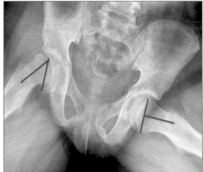

Figure 2.33.

- *AP pelvis (Figure 2.30) and frog leg lateral (Figure 2.31) showing a SUFE*
- *Figure 2.32 shows an AP Pelvis view depicting Klein's radiographic line. This line is drawn along the superior border of the femoral neck and will NOT intersect the femoral head in a child with SUFE (it does in a normal hip). The abnormality is also called a positive* **Trethowan's sign***. The left side shows a normal orientation.*
- *Figure 2.33 shows the Southwick Angle which is used to classify the degree of epiphyseal slip. It is the measurement of the femoral head-shaft ankle on the frog leg lateral. The difference between the affected and unaffected side determines the degree of slip.*
- *Other signs demonstrated by Figures 2.30–33 include epiphysiolysis (widening or lucency of the growth plate) and the metaphyseal blanch sign of Steel (blurring of the proximal femoral metaphysis due to the overlapping of the metaphysis and the posteriorly displaced epiphysis).*

TRANSIENT SYNOVITIS

BACKGROUND

This is hip pain caused by inflammation of the synovial lining of the joint. There is usually no obvious mechanism and an insidious onset. This is a DIAGNOSIS OF EXCLUSION of any other pathologies, commonly those listed in this chapter.

RADIOLOGICAL ASSESSMENT

Generally, plane radiographs do not add anything to the diagnosis however should be requested as a means of excluding other pathology within the differential diagnosis process.

KEY POINTS – HISTORY

As per all the above sections.

Specifically any recent or current coughs/colds?

KEY POINTS – CLINICAL ASSESSMENT

As per all the above section.

Generally Kocher Criteria score <2

MANAGEMENT

- If unwell or in significant pain, they may require admission for analgesia (paracetamol and NSAIDs usually suffice).
- If in doubt, admit the patient as they may need further imaging, e.g. ultrasound, to help exclude other pathology.

TOP TIPS

Remember this is a DIAGNOSIS OF EXCLUSION. Liaise with the paediatric team for them to exclude any other causes of pain.

If simple analgesic agents fail to control the pain, then consider other diagnosis.

EMERGENCY DEPARTMENT

BOAST GUIDELINES

The British Orthopaedic Association (BOA) has produced several guidelines concerning key traumatic injuries in a bid to standardise patient care. These are referred to as BOAST Guidelines (British Orthopaedic Association Standards in Trauma). They are freely available on the internet and very useful in setting out what actions should be performed when patients with key injuries present to hospital. These can be accessed at:

http://www.boa.ac.uk/publications/boa-standards-trauma-boasts/

At the time of writing, there are eleven in total. As more standards are agreed, more may be made available or current ones updated so it is important to keep up to date. They are very easy to read and provide plenty of useful advice such as what antibiotics to administer and when to refer to regional trauma centres. Should such patients present during your on call, they will be a valuable source of information.

Key ones to be aware of (and a brief summary of the key points):

BOAST 1: THE MANAGEMENT OF NECK OF FEMUR FRACTURES

The guidelines advocate early MDT team involvement, with the aim of surgery to allow the patient to fully weight bear on day 1. They highlight the need for adequate analgesia, assessment for risk of VTE and for pressure ulcers. In difficult diagnostic cases, if radiographs are equivocal, an MRI (ideally) or CT should be performed with a view to performing the surgery on the same day or the subsequent day.

BOAST 3: THE MANAGEMENT OF PELVIC FRACTURES

Major pelvic fractures may be associated with major haemorrhage. In such cases, a pelvic binder, crossed sheet or laparotomy may aid resuscitation. If there is ongoing haemorrhage, losses should be replaced with blood products and patients should be considered for open pelvic packing or embolization. There should be a high index of suspicion for urological injuries. Open fractures with wounds to buttocks, groin, rectum or genitals require a urethral catheter and bowel diversion with an end colostomy. Image transfer to appropriate specialist centres should take place within 24 hours to allow for definitive surgical planning.

BOAST 4: THE MANAGEMENT OF OPEN LOWER LIMB FRACTURES (WHICH IN PRACTICE CAN BE APPLIED TO UPPER LIMB INJURIES)

These guidelines advocate early use of antibiotic treatment. Wounds should be covered in water-soaked gauze, although should only be washed if grossly contaminated. Strict assessment and monitoring of neurovascular status and compartment syndrome should be maintained. Fractures should be reduced and immobilized to minimise soft tissue damage. There should be early multi-disciplinary involvement, typically orthopaedic and plastic surgeons.

BOAST 6: THE MANAGEMENT OF ARTERIAL INJURIES

Active haemorrhage should be controlled by direct pressure or application tourniquet, with repeated neurovascular assessment of the injured limb. Deformed limbs should be reduced, splinted and reassessed for neurovascular status. A devascularised limb needs urgent surgical exploration and will require early involvement of relevant surgical specialists e.g. vascular, orthopaedic or plastic surgeons.

BOAST 10: THE DIAGNOSIS AND MANAGEMENT OF COMPARTMENT SYNDROME

Ensure that there are repeated neurovascular assessments of the injured limb. All circumferential splints and dressings should be removed. Compartment pressure measurement can and should be performed. Urgent decompression of the compartment should be performed.

BOAST 11: THE MANAGEMENT OF SUPRACONDYLAR FRACTURES IN CHILDREN

Ensure that there are repeated neurovascular assessments of the injured limb. The majority of vascular impairments resolve with reduction of the displaced fracture; a perfused limb does not require brachial artery exploration. However, if the limb remains ischaemic after reduction, exploration of the brachial artery should be performed. In the presence of vascular compromise, surgical treatment should be performed as a matter of urgency.

OPERATING THEATRE

PREPARING A PATIENT FOR THEATRE

When in doubt, you can always assume a patient may require an operation and plan them according to the guidance below:

Almost all patients (except paediatric patients) should have:

- Full blood count.
- Urea and electrolytes.
- Group and Save (certainly obtain if long bone fractures have occurred).
- MRSA swabs.

If you are unsure what tests are needed, ask your senior. It is much easier and more efficient to get all the necessary done before the operation date as this avoids unnecessary delays on the day!

Elderly patients (generally >60 years) should have:

- ECG.
- Chest x-ray.

Any patient on anticoagulants/antiplatelet therapy

- Clotting profile.

Those with other medical conditions will require your own medical judgment. For example if someone admits to drinking large amounts of alcohol then liver function tests may be necessary.

TOP TIP

It is absolutely imperative that you follow up on the tests that have been requested to ensure that any intervention required based upon the results occurs in a timely fashion.

FASTING INSTRUCTIONS

Patients need to have been nil-by-mouth for at least 6 hours (this includes milk-based drinks) and no clear fluids for at least 2 hours prior to surgery.

Remember to document in the notes when admitting a patient to the ward AND inform the nursing team of this. If the patient is due to go home and come back for an operation in the morning, remind them not to have anything to eat or drink after midnight.

If you are not sure if the patient will require an operation or even have the operation the next day (for example due to clinical priority of other cases), there is no harm in asking them to remain fasted in any case. Prior to the trauma meeting, your senior should review all the cases and plan the list accordingly. They can always have a late breakfast!

Ensure elderly patients have IV fluid prescribed and that type 1 diabetic patients are on a sliding scale to regulate their blood sugar levels.

OPERATING THEATRE

PATIENTS ON ANTICOAGULANTS

If, for example, a patient is on warfarin and will need an operation (such as a fractured neck of femur), this should be reversed in preparation for surgery.

There are currently no reversal agents for some of the newer anticoagulants (such as rivaroxiban) or antiplatelet agents. If surgery cannot be delayed, then they should be warned about an increased risk of bleeding. Hospitals usually have their own policies on reversal of anticoagulants which you can familiarise yourself with.

Be aware of any patients with metallic heart valves or drug eluting cardiac stents as they may require discussion with your senior and/or the haematology department.

OPERATING THEATRE

PATIENTS REQUIRING EMERGENCY OPERATIONS

Although uncommon in this specialty, on occasion a patient may present who requires an emergency operation. Should this be the case, then of course your senior colleagues will be present to perform it.

For emergency referrals that are made to you out-of-hours, you may be asked to "get the patient ready" for a procedure the following day by your senior colleagues. It is best to await this confirmation before you start the process of preparing a patient for theatre.

Ensure all your investigations are complete as detailed above.

In addition to the actions described above, you should inform the on-call anaesthetic team and the theatre coordinator that there is a potential emergency case pending review by your seniors.

OPERATING
THEATRE

CONSENT FOR COMMON OPERATIONS

Generally, the consenting process should be carried out by a person experienced in the proposed procedure and able to have an in-depth discussion with the patient about alternative options, outcomes, risks and complications. As a result a senior doctor usually performs it.

However, with increasing experience, you may wish to consent patients for their upcoming operations. You should not consent a patient for any procedure that you are not familiar with or not able to discuss complications or alternative options. The consenting process is an important learning exercise and an excellent way to ensure your understanding of surgical procedures.

The commonest procedures you may consent for include:

HIP HEMIARTHROPLASTY

INDICATION

- Intracapsular neck of femur fracture

AIM OF PROCEDURE

- Pain control and mobilisation

GENERAL RISKS

- Pain, Scar, Infection, Bleeding, Swelling, Stiffness, Injury to neurovascular structures, DVT, PE, Chest infection

SPECIFIC RISKS

- Fracture
- Dislocation
- Loosening
- Leg length discrepancy
- Acetabular erosion (especially in the younger, more active patient; may do better with a total hip replacement)

OPERATING THEATRE

DYNAMIC HIP SCREW

INDICATION

- Extracapsular neck of femur fracture

AIM OF PROCEDURE

- Pain control and mobilisation

GENERAL RISKS

- Pain, Scar, Infection, Bleeding, Swelling, Stiffness, Injury to neurovascular structures, DVT, PE, Chest infection

SPECIFIC RISKS

- Fracture
- Screw cut out (tip of the screw breaking through the femoral head cortex)
- Femoral Head Collapse
- Avascular necrosis of femoral head

OPERATING
THEATRE

OPEN REDUCTION AND INTERNAL FIXATION (INCLUDING ANKLE/WRIST JOINT)

INDICATION

- Fracture of a bone (including ankle/wrist joint)

AIM OF PROCEDURE

- Fracture fixation and improvement in pain and function

GENERAL RISKS

- Pain, Scar, Infection, Bleeding, Swelling, Stiffness, Injury to neurovascular structures, DVT, PE, Chest infection

SPECIFIC RISKS

- Non union (the bone failing to heal)
- Mal union (the bone healing in a non-anatomical position)
- Delay union (the bone taking longer to heal)
- Irritation of tendons due to metalwork inserted
- Removal of metalwork
- Restricted range of movement
- Future arthritis (if involving articular surface)

OPERATING THEATRE

MANIPULATION UNDER ANAESTHESIA OF A FRACTURE/DISLOCATED JOINT

INDICATION

- Displaced, mal-aligned, dislocated or rotated fracture of a bone or joint

AIM OF PROCEDURE

- To reduce the fracture to a more anatomical position. This could be a definitive management option (e.g. a shoulder dislocation) or as a temporary procedure to allow the soft tissue to rest prior to the definitive procedure (e.g. ankle fracture-dislocation)

GENERAL RISKS

- Pain, Scar, Infection, Bleeding, Swelling, Stiffness, Injury to neurovascular structures, DVT, PE, Chest infection

SPECIFIC RISKS

- Non union (the bone failing to heal)
- Mal union (the bone healing in a non-anatomical position)
- Delay union (the bone taking longer to heal)
- Loss of position requiring further surgery

INTRAMEDULLARY NAIL INSERTION OF A LONG BONE FRACTURE

INDICATION

- Extra-articular long bone fractures (especially femur and tibia)

AIM OF PROCEDURE

- Fracture alignment and fixation

GENERAL RISKS

- Pain, Scar, Infection, Bleeding, Swelling, Stiffness, Injury to neurovascular structures, DVT, PE, Chest infection

SPECIFIC RISKS

- Non union (the bone failing to heal)
- Mal union (the bone healing in a non-anatomical position)
- Delay union (the bone taking longer to heal)
- Removal of metalwork

OPERATING THEATRE

ARTHROSCOPIC WASHOUT OF A SEPTIC JOINT

INDICATION

- Septic joint washout

AIM OF PROCEDURE

- Irrigation of a septic joint and collection of soft tissue samples

GENERAL RISKS

- Pain, Scar, Infection, Bleeding, Swelling, Stiffness, Injury to neurovascular structures, DVT, PE, Chest infection

SPECIFIC RISKS

- Persistent swelling of the affected joint
- Further surgical procedures for treatment or diagnosis

OPERATING
THEATRE

THE WARD

GENERAL PRINCIPLES

Most hospitals have dedicated orthopaedic inpatient wards where the vast majority of patients recover either pre- or post-surgery. In some cases, there may be separate wards to differentiate between patients who have undergone an elective operation (such as a joint arthroplasty) or a trauma-related operation (such as fixation of a long bone fracture). The former group are treated somewhat differently in that they generally require purely physiotherapy and early wound management, prior to being discharged more rapidly than a patient, for example, who may be elderly and recovering from a neck of femur fracture. Furthermore, segregating pre-screened post-operative elective patients from emergency post-operative patients has been shown to decrease the incidence of post-operative infections.

Despite this subtle difference in approaches, in both cases, medical care is supplemented by a group of multidisciplinary allied professionals alongside whom we should work very closely and amicably. It offers an excellent opportunity to develop your communication and management skills. It goes without saying that all allied professionals should be respected and given the same regard as we would expect to be given to ourselves. They are there to help you and not to create extra work!

THE MULTIDISCIPLINARY TEAM

ORTHOGERIATRICIANS

Almost universally now, elderly orthopaedic patients have medical input from a dedicated orthogeriatric team during daytime working hours. This is usually only for neck of femur fracture patients as this forms part of the National Hip Fracture Audit and subsequent best practice tariff payment. In some busier units, this may constitute an entire team (a consultant with their junior staff) or sometimes solely a senior clinician who regularly attends the ward to attend pre- and post-operative elderly patients. Although they are only expected to look after the elderly trauma patients (there is usually a cut off age), they are a useful source of medical advice for any other patients. You can imagine how useful this is, especially bearing in mind that the complex needs of our patients are ever increasing. It is important to anticipate and prepare for their ward rounds; ensure observations and relevant blood tests are up to date and that thromboprophylaxis and bone protection medications are prescribed if appropriate. A smooth ward round with this team is not only a chance to offer our patients expert medical input but also a fantastic opportunity to further your learning.

PHYSIOTHERAPISTS/HAND THERAPISTS

This group of allied healthcare professionals are a key ally to any orthopaedic department. These are the people who often have the more challenging job of helping our patients recover as fast as possible from their injuries and operations. Some of them may be extremely senior and may have a few useful suggestions. They may ask you to clarify post-operative instructions or confirm the weight-bearing status of certain patients; alternatively they may inform you that a patient is unable to comply with the desired post-operative instructions. When in doubt, please ask your seniors for clarification.

OCCUPATIONAL THERAPISTS

Another key ally to our department, these therapists come to assess a patient's potential needs for discharge to a safe environment. Again, they may need clarification of post-operative instructions and anticipated timelines for full mobility. When in doubt, please ask your seniors for input.

THE WARD

MULTIDISCIPLINARY TEAM (MDT) MEETINGS

These meetings happen more commonly than orthopaedic surgeons think! Although unlike other specialties, they usually do not involve the medical doctors. They tend to be related to delayed patient discharges and comprise of the patient (if appropriate) and their family, physiotherapists, occupational therapists, social workers and senior nursing staff. On occasion though, you may be asked to be present to answer medical-related questions or concerns raised. You should not feel daunted by this but preparation for such a meeting is a must! Read the patient's notes thoroughly beforehand and make sure you are aware of any post-operative complications that may have occurred. You can liaise beforehand with the involved allied professionals to ensure that you are adequately prepared and briefed for the meeting. Again, if in doubt of any aspects of the patient's care, liaise with your seniors.

THE WARD

GENERAL POST-OPERATIVE MANAGEMENT

WOUND MANAGEMENT

Unless covered by a plaster cast, patients will usefully have a visible wound covered by a dressing that was applied intra-operatively. Skin wounds tend to take around 10-14 days to heal and so during that time, appropriate measures must be taken to maintain a clean wound environment. Unless the wound is constantly oozing, the dressing has become unstuck, soiled or is completely blood stained, the wound SHOULD NOT BE disturbed (unless the post-operative notes state otherwise, e.g. in the case of a potentially contaminated injury). The more times a wound is uncovered, the higher the chance of it becoming infected. Wounds generally should be looked at once at around 5 days to ensure that all is in order and then a week later to confirm healing. If a wound does need to be redressed or looked at, this should be done using an aseptic technique and in the presence of a senior medical professional so as to minimise the exposure time. In cases of concern, a photograph using the departmental camera can be taken for future reference.

WOUND INFECTIONS

The routine assessment of post-operative wounds is not a uniform process and it is important to check with your senior colleagues whether they want the post-operative dressing to remain for 2 weeks (unless there is substantial wound ooze) or they want the wound looked at after a set number of days. Wound infections may present with subtle cellulitis around the wound edges with mild serous discharge, or at their worst with a patient that is septic, in extremis with pus oozing out of a dehisced wound.

In your routine assessment make a note of whether there is cellulitis, if the wound edges are well apposed and if there is any discharge. If there is discharge then swab it and send it off for microbiological assessment. The culture of an organism and its antibiotics sensitivities are far more likely if performed before the start of antibiotics. In the case of a surgical wound where a deeper collection is suspected an aspiration, under radiological guidance if necessary, can be performed. If the wound infection overlies a joint replacement and there is concern about an infection within the joint speak to your senior about aspiration of the joint in theatre at the earliest possible moment, and before antibiotics are commenced.

THE WARD

The key points with wound infections are:

- Get your seniors involved as soon as possible.
- Liaise with microbiology on appropriate antibiotic treatment.
- Ensure that adequate dressings are used and this may require input from tissue viability nurses if there is an area of wound breakdown. Occasionally these patients need some form of negative pressure dressing.

PLASTER CASTS

A plaster cast should be neither too tight nor too loose. Rarely after an operation will a full, circumferential plaster cast be applied (unless the procedure was a simple manipulation). Usually a partial plaster (e.g. backslab) is applied to allow and accommodate for swelling around the operative site. A patient should not be complaining of the plaster being tight and it should not be indenting the skin. If it is doing any of the above, an assessment for compartment syndrome is mandatory. Never be afraid to split or remove a plaster if you are worried it is too tight and may be causing compartment syndrome (see page 26). An operation can always be redone but the effects of a delayed or missed compartment syndrome can be devastating.

POST-OPERATIVE RADIOGRAPHS

Almost all patients require radiographs post-operatively to allow us to visualise adequacy of our surgical intervention. In most cases, the weight-bearing status or post-operative instructions are not dependent on this radiograph and so the rehabilitation process can start without this. However in some cases, decisions may be made after this has been done. The patient should only be sent for these radiographs if they are safe to leave the ward and go to the radiology department; if they are not then the radiograph should be delayed. Always get your seniors to review the radiographs and document this in the patient notes, along with any changes to the post-operative regimen related to this.

THE WARD

WARD MANAGEMENT OF PATIENTS WITH COMMON INJURIES

PATIENTS WITH A HIP FRACTURE

The management of patients with a hip fracture will take up most of your time when providing ward-level patient care. These patients are generally quite elderly and frail. The myriad of medical conditions they have make them quite complex to manage and the additional effect of their surgery further complicates their care. There are useful guidelines from NICE and the BOA which should be read if you are starting a job in trauma and orthopaedics. These guidelines are very helpful in understanding the basics of management. They often form the basis of local patient pathways that you may find useful for patients with a hip fracture.

Pre-operative ward level care often lasts no longer than 24 hours because of the drive to operate on these patients as soon as possible. There is a strong evidence base that underlines that early surgery improves a patient's relative risk of death. There are a few key points to consider prior to surgery when these patients are on the ward:

- Ensure they have adequate analgesia prescribed.
- Make sure that IV fluids are prescribed.
- For patients that are diabetic start a sliding scale if they are fasting.
- Adhere to your local thromboprophylaxis protocols.
- Liaise with anaesthetists and orthogeriatricians at an early stage.

One of the commonest causes of delay to surgery is because patients are anti-coagulated and there is confusion about how to manage this peri-operatively. Speak to your on-call haematologist at the earliest possible stage. There are a number of different blood thinning agents and generally they should not delay time to surgery. A few examples include:

- Patients on 75mg aspirin daily are safe to have surgery.
- Patients on clopidogrel can generally have platelets at induction of anaesthesia.
- Patients on warfarin for atrial fibrillation can generally be given Vitamin K orally and have their INR checked after 6 hours. If their INR is less than 1.5 than they can have their surgery.
- Patients with a mechanical heart valve or a pulmonary embolism on warfarin may need a heparin infusion. Speak to haematology at the earliest possible opportunity to ensure that this is set up quickly so that surgery is not delayed.

THE WARD

The post-operative management of these patients should start with reading the operation note. Standard measures such as post-operative blood tests, thromboprophylaxis and check x-rays may be the norm, however referring to the operation notes is extremely important as there may be patient-specific assessments or rehabilitation (weight-bearing status) that are required.

Post-operative anaemia is associated with poor functional outcomes and mortality rates, however there is growing consensus that transfusion should be spared for anaemic patients who are symptomatic or in patients whose haemoglobin is less than 80g/dl. Ensure that post-operative analgesia is adequate. Check with nursing staff when patients last opened their bowels as constipation and post-operative ileus are commonplace amongst these patients. Look out for signs of delirium and sepsis, and closely liaise with your orthogeriatrics team in the medical management of these patients.

PATIENTS WITH A WRIST FRACTURE

Patients with upper limb fractures are generally ambulatory post-surgery and need not stay in hospital longer than a day. Prior to discharge a neurological assessment of the affected limb should be performed and documented. The cast should be assessed to make sure it's not too tight. Provided that these assessments are satisfactory and that the patient is clinically stable they may be discharged. In elderly, frail patients, especially those who use a walking aid on the injured side, there may be a need for longer inpatient stay and convalescence as they may not be safe for early discharge.

PATIENTS WITH AN ANKLE FRACTURE

Commonly, when these patients are admitted for surgery in the aftermath of their injury, their ankle swells up. Closing the surgical wound on a swollen ankle can be quite problematic and as a result there is a preference to elevate these limbs for 5-7 days to allow the ankle swelling to settle. Keep a close eye on these patients and make sure they have a Braun frame (or a few pillows) under their ankle to help the swelling settle. In the post-operative period ensure that their weight-bearing status is adhered to upon discharge and that appropriate thromboprophylaxis is prescribed for patients upon discharge. For patients who have non-absorbable stitches in their wound, planned follow up must be by at least 2 weeks so the sutures can be removed.

THE WARD

PATIENTS WITH TIBIAL SHAFT FRACTURES

The main concern with these patients is that pre- or post-operatively they may develop a compartment syndrome. Regular limb observations can normally be performed by nursing staff, however it is important to ensure that an immediate assessment is performed if concern is raised. The most important sign is pain out of proportion with the presenting injury which is associated with worse pain on passive stretch of the muscle compartment affected. Paraesthesia, paralysis and an absent pulse are late signs. Discussion with a senior should occur at the earliest opportunity and if there is uncertainty based on clinical assessment or in the case of an unconscious patient then compartment pressures should be measured.

PAEDIATRIC PATIENTS

One of the aspects of orthopaedics that is often very new and novel to junior doctors starting their training is the fact that we have paediatric patients. It's important to recognise that these patients are very different from adults and their care has to be tailored to their needs. There are a few things not to forget when managing paediatric patients on the ward:

- You are treating a vulnerable, scared child and vulnerable, scared parents. Be kind. Keep the parents up to date on treatment on a regular basis.

- Don't be afraid to speak to your seniors or the paediatrics team if the child seems unwell or you have concerns regarding their wellbeing and safety.

- In the pre-operative assessment of these patients blood tests are often required. If your venepuncture and venous cannulation skills are not up to the standard required to bleed or get venous access from a toddler, ask a paediatrician for help. Do not subject a child to repeated attempts to get blood.

THE WARD

THE CLINIC

FRACTURE CLINIC

You may have the opportunity to attend fracture clinic and it's important to have an approach to manage patients effectively and efficiently.

Always refer to the last correspondence prior to seeing the patient. A surgical operation note, discharge letter or clinic letter will provide key information on the patient's injury, the treatment they have received and what is required at the clinic review. Patients commonly need an x-ray, a change of plaster or a wound review and if you can arrange these in advance of seeing the patient it will allow the assessment to be performed fluently.

Wound assessments are normally done in the plaster room, not the clinic room. Ensure you have the wound care pack and new dressings at hand before removing any dressings if you are doing it yourself. Always ensure you have checked whether absorbable or non-absorbable sutures were used and have a plan about when the latter need to be removed.

For patients who are attending clinic for the first time and have a backslab on that needs to be converted to a full cast, make an effort to assess the limb clinically when they are having a change of plaster to see whether there is any injury to the skin or a plastic deformity of the limb. Use this time to perform a neurovascular assessment of the limb as well.

An important part of the assessment process involves the documentation of your assessment in the clinical notes and also your dictation for the clinical letter that is sent out to the GP. Be clear in your dictation and speak slowly. Make sure you have stated the patient's name, hospital number and date of birth at the start of each letter. Your senior colleagues may have a specific format they prefer for the letter layout, however presented below is an example of what is expected. Remember to keep your letters short and to the point.

10.03.2017

Dear Doctor,

Re: John Smith, DOB 01/01/1920, Hospital Number X12345

Injury: Weber B Ankle Fracture 01.01.2017

Surgery: Open reduction and internal fixation 02.01.2017

Current management plan: Mobilise full weight bearing and discharge to physiotherapy

First paragraph: History of injury and current patient progress

Second paragraph: Clinical and radiological assessment in the clinic today

Final Paragraph: Plan initiated in the clinic today and follow up plan.

Yours sincerely,

Dr Peter Smith, MBBS BSc

CT1 Trauma and Orthopaedics

VIRTUAL FRACTURE CLINIC (VFC)

It's unlikely that as a junior grade doctor you will be directly involved in the running of the VFC but it's worth understanding what it is. The VFC involves a senior doctor (usually a consultant) reviewing the clinical notes and x-rays of patients referred from ED for a fracture clinic appointment. A decision is made on whether a fracture clinic review is required, and if it is, which fracture clinic would be appropriate for the patient to attend. A member of the team usually calls patients after the VFC to inform them about the plan.

Most departments have fracture management pathways that guide ED staff on how patients should be managed. This usually includes which patients need to be referred to the on-call orthopaedic team and which patients can be referred into the VFC system. Find out about these pathways early in your job as it will help you triage many of the referrals you receive.

THE CLINIC

THE PLASTER ROOM

The plaster room is where patients go to have plaster casts/backslabs changed or applied. Assessment of wounds can also usually be performed in the plaster room and nursing staff or plaster technicians are generally able to help with wound care and removal of sutures. The plaster room may also house the common splints and braces.

When you are in clinic you will be in and out of the plaster room assessing patients. Be clear with your written instructions to the staff in the plaster room. State what level you want the cast applied to, what material of cast you want to use and what position you want the limb to be in. For lower limb plasters also be clear on the weight bearing status of the patient. If you have free time during your placement spend a few mornings in the plaster room as this is quite a useful experience to learn basic plastering techniques.

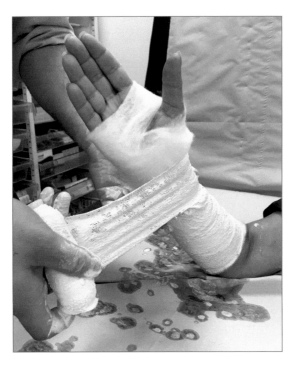

Fig 5.1. The application of an upper limb plaster in the plaster room

THE CLINIC

ADMITTING PATIENTS FROM CLINIC

Patients seen in fracture clinic are often required to undergo surgical management of their fractures. These patients may either be admitted straight to a ward for surgery or they may come back on a specific day for surgery (such cases are commonly termed 'TCI' or 'To come in'). Either way these patients need to have a full medical history taken, a comprehensive clinical examination performed and appropriate pre-operative investigations organised. As a junior doctor in trauma and orthopaedics, this is something you will be called on to do.

The history taking should focus on the injury being treated but there should also be a full past medical history, medication, allergy and social history taken. It's important to know all about these aspects of the patient's history because it will also be your responsibility to discuss the case with an anaesthetist. Furthermore, if a patient is on any anticoagulation therapy or has a latex allergy and these facts are not picked up, it could result in serious harm coming to the patient. In terms of pre-operative tests, these need to be tailored to the patient and the procedure being performed but consider the need for the following:

- Blood tests: clotting, full blood count, renal function and a Group & Save.
- ECG.
- MRSA swabs (more useful for TCI patients).
- Ask a ward clerk to request the patients entire clinical notes if not available.
- Chest x-ray.
- Urine dipstick.

Consent for some common orthopaedic procedures has been introduced in the previous chapter, but bear in mind unless you have seen the operation being proposed and understand the steps involved and the risks associated with it well, leave this to a more senior colleague. Speak to your trauma coordinator and bed manager to inform them of the admission and to try and organise a hospital bed. Also make sure you discuss the case with an anaesthetist so that further assessments (echocardiogram/lung function tests) can be organised if they are felt to be necessary.

THE CLINIC

PROCEDURES

HAEMATOMA BLOCK USING LOCAL ANAESTHETIC

This is commonly used for closed manipulation of wrist fractures and can be the sole analgesic agent required to perform the reduction.

PREPARATION/EQUIPMENT

10ml sterile syringe.

x 2 hypodermic needles (sterile).

5-10ml Local anaesthetic (either lidocaine (fast and short acting agent) alone or combination of lidocaine and bupivacaine (prolonged action).

TECHNIQUE

- Ensure that the area is clean and dry.
- Look and feel for the fracture on the dorsum (back) of the wrist – this will feel like a bump.
- There are no neurovascular structures on the dorsum of the wrist and hence it is a good access point to inject the local anaesthetic.
- Draw up your local anaesthetic.
- Insert the needle and syringe at an angle of around 30 degrees to the skin to the region of the fracture.

Figure 6.1. Delivery of haematoma block.

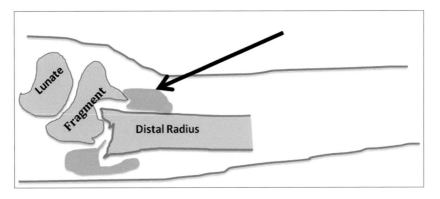

- Aspirate to ensure you get a blood flashback – this is the haematoma associated with the fracture and confirms that you are in the correct area.
- Slowly inject the local anaesthetic.

MANIPULATION AND REDUCTION OF DORSALLY DISPLACED WRIST FRACTURES

ALWAYS assess neurovascular status both pre- and post-manipulation

PREPARATION/EQUIPMENT

Plaster trolley set up and to hand.

You will typically need 2 assistants. Two people are required to perform the reduction and 1 to apply the plaster.

TECHNIQUE

- Performed under either regional anaesthesia (such as haematoma block), IV sedation (typically midazolam or morphine) or entonox gas.
- An assistant stands next to the patient's head and holds the distal humerus above the elbow, keeping the joint flexed at 90 degrees. Their role is to provide counter-traction.
- The person doing the reduction stands in front and facing the assistant, and controls the distal fragment, holding the hand with both hands, placing his thumbs over the dorsal surface of the distal fragment.

COMMON REDUCTION MANOEUVRE FOR A DORSALLY DISPLACED FRACTURE

- Increase the deformity, apply traction in this hyperextended position, translate it distally until it can be 'hooked over' the proximal fragment, reduce the fragment to its acceptable position by flexing it and applying some ulna deviation.
- Immobilise the hand with a plaster on the dorsal side.

PROCEDURES

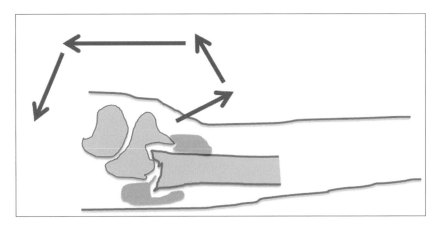

Figure 6.2. Common reduction manoeuvre for a dorsally displaced fracture.

- In the reduced position, a third person (second assistant) applies the plaster backslab on the dorsal aspect of the wrist as this will act as a 'block' to stop the fragment slipping back to its injury position.

TOP TIP

In the case of a volar displaced fracture (e.g. Smith's type fracture), the backslab should be placed on the volar aspect of the wrist to block displacement.

PROCEDURES

MANIPULATION AND REDUCTION OF ANKLE FRACTURES

ALWAYS assess neurovascular status both pre- and post-manipulation

PREPARATION/EQUIPMENT

This is typically done under IV sedation so you usually need to liaise with the ED staff, who will often monitor the patient during their reduction.

Plaster trolley set up and to hand.

You will typically need 2 assistants. Two people are required to perform the reduction and 1 to apply the plaster.

TECHNIQUE

- Check both the AP and lateral radiographs to orientate yourself with the fracture pattern and thus in which direction the reduction needs to be performed (i.e. which direction has the talus moved; the direction of your reduction should aim to move the talus to its natural position, thus reducing the lateral and/or medial malleolus simultaneously).
- The patient should be lying supine on a trolley. One assistant stands at the level of the pelvis, facing the end of the bed. They hold the hip and knee flexed at 90 degree angles. By flexing the knee, the Achilles tendon relaxes and thus the surgeon can control and manipulate the distal fracture with more ease.
- The person doing the reduction, grasps the calcaneum with one hand and, according to the direction of the displacement, moves it in the appropriate plane to achieve the reduction. With their other hand, they can apply counter traction to the distal tibia to aid reduction.
- A third person then applies the plaster backslab. It is sometimes necessary for the reduction to be released in order to position the plaster. If this is the case, then whilst the plaster is still soft and malleable, the same reduction technique is performed until the plaster has hardened.

PROCEDURES

TOP TIPS

It is often easier to apply wool prior to reducing the fracture. You will find that trying to hold a reduced fracture in the correct position while then applying a wool dressing can be very awkward and can often lead to you losing your reduction.

The ankle should be in a neutral position in the plaster; it commonly drifts into equinus so you must ensure that the position is maintained until the plaster has fully set.

MANIPULATION AND REDUCTION OF SHOULDER DISLOCATIONS

ALWAYS assess neurovascular status both pre- and post-manipulation

PREPARATION/EQUIPMENT

You will often require assistants.

Commonly performed under intravenous anaesthesia, so you will need to liaise closely with the ED registrar or anaesthetist.

There are numerous described methods on how to reduce a dislocated shoulder, the commonest of which are:

1. TRACTION/COUNTER TRACTION METHOD (ADAPTED FROM THE HIPPOCRATIC MANOEUVRE)

- This is a two person technique.
- Pass a sheet under the patient's axilla on the affected side. The two ends, making a U shape around the axilla, are then held by an assistant.
- Stand facing the patient on the affected side and grasp the distal wrist or forearm.
- With the arm in a degree of abduction, apply longitudinal traction, whilst the assistant applies counter traction by pulling the sheet in the opposite direction to the surgeon's pull. Sometimes, a little rotation during traction helps unhinge the humeral head and reduce the joint.

2. KOCHER TECHNIQUE

- The patient may be supine or sitting up at 45 degrees.
- Flex the elbow in the affected limb to 90 degrees at the elbow.
- Keeping the elbow adducted against the body, hold the elbow in one hand and the patient's wrist in the other.
- Slowly externally rotate between 70 degrees to 85 degrees until resistance is felt. Then flex (lift forwards) the externally rotated upper arm and internally rotate the shoulder (i.e. bring the patient's hand that you are holding towards their opposite shoulder). The humeral head should now slip back into the glenoid fossa.

PROCEDURES

3. STIMSON TECHNIQUE

- The patient lies prone on a bed with the affected arm hanging down in forward flexion.
- Place a sandbag under the clavicle on the affected side and apply a weight (usually not more than 10lb) to the wrist on the affected side.
- The weight must hang above the ground and not touch the floor. The muscles eventually relax and the joint normally reduces spontaneously.

PROCEDURES

APPLICATION OF SKIN TRACTION

ALWAYS assess neurovascular status both pre- and post-manipulation

This is useful in patients who have suffered femoral fractures (including neck of femur fractures) as a method of reducing pain due to muscle spasm whilst maintaining the limb in a position of comfort and rest. It may also reduce further soft tissue injury and restore blood flow and nerve function.

PREPARATION/EQUIPMENT

Ensure that the patient is in an appropriate bed that can accommodate the traction gallows.

Check the skin for abrasions/bruises.

TECHNIQUE

- Open the skin extension set and whilst applying and maintaining traction to the limb, use the bandage provided in the set to wrap the traction arms around the affected limb.
- Leave sufficient room between the patient's foot and the end of the skin extension.
- Apply an appropriate weight (not more than 10% of the patient's body weight) to the hanging strings. Ensure that the weights hang freely above the ground and are not obstructed.
- Elevate the foot of the bed.

TOP TIP

Some of the traction sets may have arms with an adhesive backing. If the skin is not very thin or frail, you can stick this on the skin. However if there is any concern, simply use the bandage to wrap it around the limb.

PROCEDURES

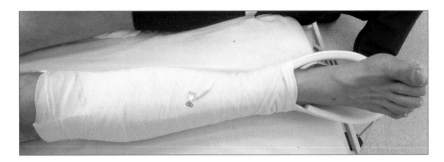

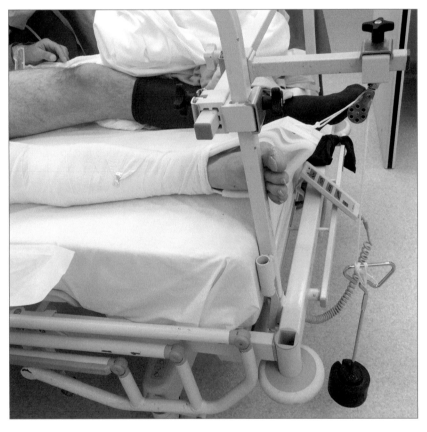

Fig 6.3a&b. The application of lower
limb skin traction

RING/DIGITAL BLOCK

ALWAYS assess neurovascular status both pre- and post-manipulation

This is useful for phalangeal dislocations in the hand or foot. While performing these blocks, it is key to remember that each digit is innovated by 4 nerves; 2 palmar nerves and 2 dorsal nerves in the upper limb, and 2 dorsal nerves and 2 plantar nerves in the lower limb.

PREPARATION/EQUIPMENT

10ml sterile syringe.

x 2 hypodermic needles (sterile).

5-10ml Local anaesthetic (either lidocaine (fast and short acting agent) alone or combination of lidocaine and bupivacaine (prolonged action).

TECHNIQUE

- Ensure that the correct digit is identified.
- Make sure the area is clean.
- Insert the needle at the level of the webspace on the dorsal side. Aim for the midline of the phalanx, just to either side of the tendon.
- Push the needle straight down until you hit the bone. Then move slightly to the side until you just come off the bony edge. Aspirate to ensure you are not in a vessel and then inject 3-5mls local anaesthetic.
- With the needle still in the skin, work your way back round the dorsal aspect of the bone until you drop down the other side of the bone. Aspirate to ensure you are not in a vessel and then inject 3-5mls local anaesthetic.

TOP TIP

NEVER use local anaesthetic containing adrenaline for this procedure as it may cause digital ischaemia.

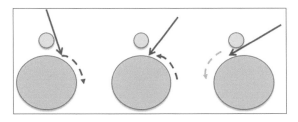

Figure 6.4. Steps for performing digital block.

- *Needle (red arrow)*
- *Tendon (yellow circle)*
- *Phalanx (grey circle)*

PROCEDURES

KNEE ASPIRATION

Never aspirate a knee with a prosthesis in situ in the accident and emergency department! This should be done in theatre.

The knee is the commonest joint to be aspirated. Usually the patient will either have their knee slightly flexed or completely straight.

PREPARATION/EQUIPMENT

Skin cleansing solution.

10ml local anaesthetic (optional).

10ml sterile syringe.

Wide bore needle (for example a 16 gauge white needle).

Sticky plaster.

Specimen bottle/blood culture bottles.

TECHNIQUE

If there is a large swelling, it makes the procedure much easier.

Feel for the outline border of the patella. If the effusion is intra-articular, this will ALWAYS be palpable.

There are several entry points that can be used in order to access the knee as shown in Figure 6.5:

1. Lateral to patella tendon.
2. Medial to patella tendon.
3. Superolateral to patella.
4. Superomedial to patella.

- Select the entry point you will use; you can prod the area with your finger and thus ensure the effusion lies beneath it. You can mark the area with a marker if you wish.
- Prep the skin with the cleansing solution.
- If using local anaesthetic, insert the needle through the skin and advance in the SAME direction you would to aspirate the fluid. Inject local anaesthetic into the soft tissue, before you enter the joint. Withdraw the syringe.

PROCEDURES

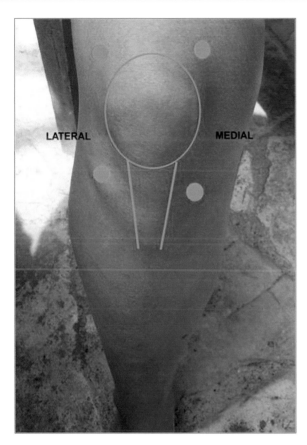

Figure 6.5. There are 4 main entry points that can be used in order to access the knee. These lie lateral to patella tendon, medial to patella tendon, superolateral to patella and superomedial to patella.

- Using the white needle (wide bore) attached to the 10ml syringe, insert into the knee joint until you are aspirating fluid.
- Once the syringe is filled, detach the needle leaving it in situ whilst you empty the syringe into the specimen bottle. Reattach the syringe and keep aspirating all the fluid.
- Once finished, apply sticky plaster to entry point.

TOP TIP:

If you cannot feel the patella border because of swelling anterior to the bone, then this is a pre-patella bursitis rather than an effusion.

Be wary of aspirating a knee through cellulitic skin; either select an alternate entry point or ask your senior for advice.

PROCEDURES

INDEX